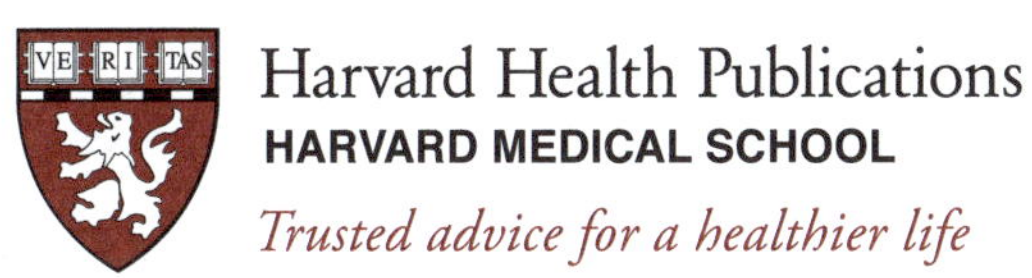

Dear Reader,

Joint pain throbs. It aches. Quite likely, it makes you think twice about everyday tasks and pleasures like going for a brisk walk, lifting your grandchild or some grocery bags, chasing a tennis ball across the court, or driving a golf ball down the fairway. Sharp reminders of your limitations occur practically every time you move.

Very often, the culprits behind joint pain are osteoarthritis, old injuries, repetitive or overly forceful movements during sports or work, posture problems, aging, or inactivity. Ignoring the pain won't make it go away. Nor will avoiding all motions that spark discomfort. In fact, limiting your movements can weaken muscles, compounding joint trouble, and affect your posture, setting off a cascade of further problems. And while pain relievers and cold or hot packs may offer quick relief, fixes like these are merely temporary.

By contrast, the right set of exercises can provide a long-lasting way to tame ankle, knee, hip, or shoulder pain. Practiced regularly, the workouts in this report might permit you to postpone—or even avoid—surgery on a problem joint that has been worsening for years, by strengthening key supportive muscles and restoring flexibility. Over time, you may find that limitations you've learned to work around will begin to ease. Tasks and opportunities for fun that you've weeded out of your routine by necessity may come back into reach, too.

Beyond the benefits to your joints, becoming more active can help you stay independent long into your later years. Regular activity is good for your heart and sharpens the mind. It nudges blood pressure down and morale up, eases stress, and keeps off unwanted pounds. Perhaps most importantly, it lessens your risk of dying prematurely. All of this can be achieved at a comfortable pace and very low cost in money or time—in fact, this report will show you how to fold many activities into your daily routine.

So select the specific workout you need. Check our safety tips, and then get started. We've combined our expertise in physical medicine and rehabilitation as well as personal training to prescribe gentle, effective warm-ups, stretches, and strengthening moves that will help you regain flexibility and build up supportive muscles. For avid golf and tennis players, or office athletes wincing from work-related repetitive motions, we've written a special section on wrists and elbows to get you back in the game.

Sincerely,

Edward M. Phillips, M.D.	Josie Gardiner	Joy Prouty
Medical Editor	*Master Trainer*	*Master Trainer*

Taking the first steps

Maybe you love to exercise. Or maybe you don't. Either way, you don't need to let joint pain stand between you and one of the most healthful activities known to mankind. In fact, the right exercises can help you control the pain. Regular exercise not only helps maintain joint function, but also reduces stiffness, pain, and fatigue. And that's in addition to a whole host of benefits for your heart, lungs, bones, muscles, and even mood.

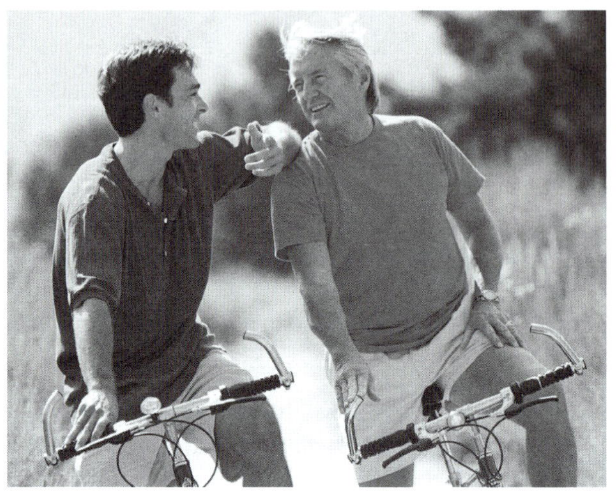

Although it might seem that exercising would aggravate aching joints, this is simply not the case. Joints tend to be more painful when they are left idle.

Thinkstock

This Special Health Report will show you how to exercise each of the major joints safely and how to set a course toward a healthier life by pairing gentle, targeted joint workouts with a simple walking plan that could add years to your life while changing it for the better. Don't let joint pain hold you back any longer.

Why exercise helps joints

Although it might seem that exercising would aggravate aching joints, this is simply not the case. Joints tend to be more painful when they are left idle. Some basic information about joints helps explain why.

A joint's structure—whether a hinge, pivot, ball-in-socket, or other formation—allows movement in many directions. Inside the joint, cartilage cushions the intersections between bones and absorbs synovial fluid, a lubricant that helps protect bones from being worn away over time by friction. Ligaments made of strong, usually inelastic tissue bind and stabilize joints. Stretchy cords of tissue called tendons tether muscle to bone and cartilage. The muscles attach to tendons, which tug on bones, allowing the body to walk and jump, dance and run—that is, to move in any way you choose.

Exercise can actually help to relieve joint pain in multiple ways.

- It increases the strength and flexibility of the muscles and connective tissue surrounding the joints. When thigh muscles are stronger, for example, they can help support the knee, thus relieving some of the pressure on that joint.
- Exercise relieves stiffness, which itself can be painful. The body is made to move. When not exercised, the tendons, muscles, and ligaments quickly shorten and tense up. But exercise—and stretching afterward—can help reduce stiffness and help preserve range of motion in a joint.
- It boosts production of synovial fluid, the lubricant inside the joints. Synovial fluid helps to bring oxygen and nutrients into joints. Thus, exercise helps keep your joints "well oiled."
- It increases production of natural compounds in the body that help tamp down pain. In other words, without exercise, you are more sensitive to every twinge. With it, you have a measure of natural pain protection.
- It helps you keep your weight under control, which can help relieve pressure in weight-bearing joints, such as your hips, knees, and ankles.

If all this isn't enough, consider the following: exercise also enhances the production of natural chemicals in the brain that help boost your mood. You'll feel happier—in addition to feeling better.

Beyond joint pain relief: Why exercise?

Why should you exercise, particularly if it prompts twinges or outright pain in your joints? Put simply, staying active helps you feel, think, and look better. Regular exercise can take a load off aching joints by strengthening muscles and chiseling away excess fat while easing swelling and pain. It allows some people to cut back on medications they take, such as drugs for high blood pressure or diabetes. And that can ease unwelcome side effects and save money.

Strong evidence from thousands of studies shows that engaging in regular exercise

- tacks years on to your life
- lowers your risks for early death, heart disease, stroke, type 2 diabetes, high blood pressure, high cholesterol, and metabolic syndrome (a complex problem that increases the risk for stroke, doubles risk for heart disease, and quintuples risk for diabetes by blending three or more of the following factors: high blood pressure, high triglycerides, low HDL cholesterol, a large waistline, and difficulty regulating blood sugar)
- helps keep your heart healthy by striking a better balance of blood lipids (HDL, LDL, and triglycerides), which prevents plaque buildup; helping arteries stay resilient despite aging; bumping up the number of blood vessels feeding the heart; reducing inflammation; and discouraging the formation of blood clots that can block coronary arteries
- lessens the likelihood of getting colon and breast cancers
- helps keep you from gaining weight
- helps prevent falls that can lead to debilitating fractures and loss of independence
- may help with weight loss (and maintaining weight loss) when combined with the proper diet; weight loss, in turn, may help slow, or even reverse, knee problems
- strengthens muscles, lungs, and heart
- eases depression
- boosts mental sharpness in older adults.

Emerging evidence suggests that regular exercise also

- improves functional abilities in older adults—that is, being able to walk up stairs or through a store, heft groceries, rise from a chair without help, and perform a multitude of other activities that permit independence or bring joy to our lives
- helps lessen abdominal obesity, which plays a role in many serious ailments, including heart disease, diabetes, and stroke
- boosts bone density (provided the exercises are weight-bearing, meaning that they work against gravity)
- lowers risk for hip fractures
- leads to better sleep
- lowers risks for lung and endometrial cancer.

How much exercise should you aim for?

The Physical Activity Guidelines from the U.S. Department of Health and Human Services urge all adults—including people with various disabilities—to meet the following targets for weekly exercise:

- Accumulate a weekly total of 150 minutes or more of moderate-intensity aerobic activity, or 75 minutes or more of vigorous activity, or an equivalent mix of the two, spread throughout the week. One way to attain this is by engaging in 30 minutes of physical activity per day, five days a week, as the American College of Sports Medicine and the American Heart Association recommend in collaborative guidelines. Or you can tot up your weekly time in exercise sessions of various lengths throughout the week. Activity should last at least five to 10 minutes at a time, with 10 minutes of vigorous activity equaling approximately 20 minutes of moderate activity. (How can you gauge whether exercise is moderate or vigorous? When doing moderate activity, you can talk, but not sing; during vigorous activity, you can say only a few words without pausing to breathe.)
- Aim for two sessions a week of strength exercises focused on the legs, hips, back, abdomen, chest, shoulders, and arms.
- If you're an older adult or otherwise at risk of falling, you should also do balance exercises.

Such a program—with 150 minutes of moderate exercise a week at its core—is sufficient to gain all the health benefits described in "Beyond joint pain relief: Why exercise?" above. However, doubling your weekly exercise time—to 300 minutes of moderate aerobic activity, or 150 minutes of vigorous activity—boosts health benefits even more.

Are you shaking your head at the thought of doing this much activity? That's not unlikely, especially

The dangers of sitting

When you're in pain, it may be hard to make yourself get up and move. But consider this: A growing body of evidence suggests that spending too many hours sitting is hazardous to your health. Habitual inactivity raises risks for obesity, diabetes, cardiovascular disease, deep-vein thrombosis, and metabolic syndrome.

Researchers aren't sure why prolonged sitting has such negative health consequences. But one possible explanation is that it relaxes your largest muscles. When muscles relax, they take up very little glucose from the blood, raising your risk of type 2 diabetes. In addition, the enzymes that break down blood fats (triglycerides) plummet, causing levels of the "good" cholesterol, HDL, to fall, too. The result? Higher risk of heart disease.

Sitting can also increase pain. Even if you're reasonably active, hours of sitting—whether reading a book, working on the computer, or watching TV—tighten the hip flexor and hamstring muscles and stiffen the joints themselves. Overly tight hip flexors and hamstrings affect gait and balance, making activities like walking harder and perhaps even setting you up for a fall. Plus, tight hip flexors and hamstrings may contribute to lower back pain and knee stiffness, scourges that many people suffer with every day.

Given the research, breaking up long blocks of sitting to flex your muscles seems like a wise move for all of us, so try to build more activity into your day. Take your phone calls standing up. Try an adjustable standing desk for your computer. Instead of sitting in an armchair while watching TV, sit on a stability ball, which makes you use your muscles to stay upright. And, yes, do our joint pain relief exercises.

if joint pain has been slowing you down. Pain often provides a seemingly ironclad excuse to pare back activities. But by letting joint pain sideline you, you squelch many joys in life. Still worse, you compromise your health, well-being, and independence, and you become vulnerable to the many problems associated with a sedentary lifestyle (see "The dangers of sitting," above). Just remember that any amount of exercise beats none. Try to do as much as possible. Even short bursts of activity (five minutes of walking several times a day to help you build endurance) are a good first step toward meeting a bigger goal.

Safety first

While it's tempting to flip right to the workout section, it's best to think about safety first. The goal of this report is to ease pain and prevent injuries, not raise the odds of both. Start with the list of conditions that should prompt you to call a doctor for advice. Then read the tips in this section aimed at helping you work out safely and effectively. After that, you'll be ready to get started.

Do you need to see a doctor?

Any doctor will tell you exercise is essential for a healthy life. But are the exercises we're recommending safe for *you*? Generally, light to moderate exercise is safe for healthy adults. Almost anyone—healthy or not—can safely take up walking. But before starting the workouts in this report, it's best to check with your doctor if

- your joints are hot, red, or swollen, particularly if you aren't usually active
- you have a chronic or unstable health condition, such as heart disease or several risk factors for heart disease, asthma or another respiratory ailment, high blood pressure, osteoporosis, or diabetes.

You may also want to use a helpful tool developed by the Canadian Society for Exercise Physiology. Called the Physical Activity Readiness Questionnaire (PAR-Q), this set of questions can help you determine whether you should talk to a doctor before embarking on or ramping up an exercise program. You can find it at www.health.harvard.edu/PAR-Q.

If you do need to speak to your doctor, ask if you can follow the program described in specific joint workouts in this report. If you're not currently exercising, discuss our proposed walking plan, too. Your doctor may feel these workouts are fine as long as you start gradually and build up slowly, or may want to modify the program to make it safer for you.

Warning signs

Call a doctor for advice if you experience any of these warning signs during or after exercise:

- ✔ sudden, sharp, or intense pain
- ✔ pain lasting one or two weeks (as distinct from delayed-onset muscle soreness, a normal response to taxing your muscles that usually peaks 24 to 48 hours after a workout and gradually abates)
- ✔ dizziness; faintness; chest pain, pressure, heaviness, or tightness; or significant or persistent shortness of breath
- ✔ in hot, humid weather: headache, dizziness, nausea, faintness, cramps, or palpitations, which are the likely signs of overheating.

If necessary, your doctor can refer you to a physiatrist, physical therapist, or another health care specialist like a cardiologist or rheumatologist for further evaluation.

Fitness professionals

Occasionally, a doctor may recommend working out with the supervision of an exercise physiologist, physical therapist, experienced personal trainer, or another certified fitness professional.

Exercise physiologists are health professionals who have completed at least a bachelor's degree in exercise science, physiology, or kinesiology. Some concentrate on research, while others design exercise programs for people with chronic ailments, including joint pain. Look for one who also holds a master's degree and is certified by the American College of Sports Medicine (ACSM) as a registered clinical exercise physiologist (RCEP).

Physiatrists, also known as rehabilitation physicians, are board-certified medical doctors who specialize in treating nerve, muscle, and bone conditions that affect movement. Knee or shoulder injuries, debilitating arthritis or obesity, stroke, back problems, and repetitive stress injuries are a few examples. A physiatrist can tailor an exercise prescription to enhance recovery after surgery or an injury, or to help you work out with limitations posed by pain or limited movement. He or she can also tell you whether certain types of exercise will be helpful or harmful given your specific health history.

Physical therapists help restore abilities to people with health conditions or injuries affecting muscles, joints, bones, or nerves. Their expertise can be valuable if, for instance, you have suffered a lingering sprain or are recovering from a heart attack or hip replacement. Some specialize in cardiopulmonary rehabilitation, orthopedics, sports medicine, geriatrics, or other areas. Physical therapists must graduate from an accredited physical therapy program, which most often offers a doctoral degree. In addition, they must pass a national exam given by the Federation of State Boards of Physical Therapy and be licensed by their state. Specialists complete advanced training and additional national exams to become board certified.

Physical therapy assistants provide physical therapy services under the supervision of a physical therapist; they must complete a two-year associate's degree, pass a national exam, and, in most states, be licensed.

Personal trainers are fitness specialists who can help ensure that you're doing exercises properly. While encouraging and motivating you, they can teach new skills, fine-tune your form, change up routines to beat boredom, and safely push you to the next level. No nationwide licensing requirements exist for personal trainers, although standards for the accrediting fitness organizations that train them have been set by the National Commission for Certifying Agencies. Two well-respected organizations that offer programs of study for personal trainers are the American College of Sports Medicine (ACSM) and the American Council on Exercise (ACE); others include the National Council on Strength and Fitness (NCSF), the National Strength and Conditioning Association (NSCA), and the National Academy of Sports Medicine (NASM). All fitness organizations have different requirements for training and expertise. Some trainers specialize in working with particular populations—for example, older adults or athletes—and may have taken courses and possibly certifying exams in these areas.

15 tips for safe exercise

Exercise is so good for you that doctors are starting to write prescriptions for it. However, it's important to follow certain safety guidelines.

Six all-around exercise safety tips

Whatever kind of exercise you choose to do, following these general tips can help you protect yourself from injury and illness.

- **Warm up properly.** Allot several minutes for this before a workout.
- **Boost your activity level gradually over time.** Start slowly, building up gradually over time. If you stop exercising for a while, don't force yourself to resume at your previous level. Drop back if necessary by doing fewer repetitions or sets, then build back up.
- **Pay attention to your body.** Don't exercise when you're sick or feeling overly fatigued. Fatigue often leads to injuries.
- **Avoid overtraining.** Follow the exercise guidelines. Training too hard or too often can cause overuse injuries like stress fractures, stiff or sore joints and muscles, and inflamed tendons and ligaments.

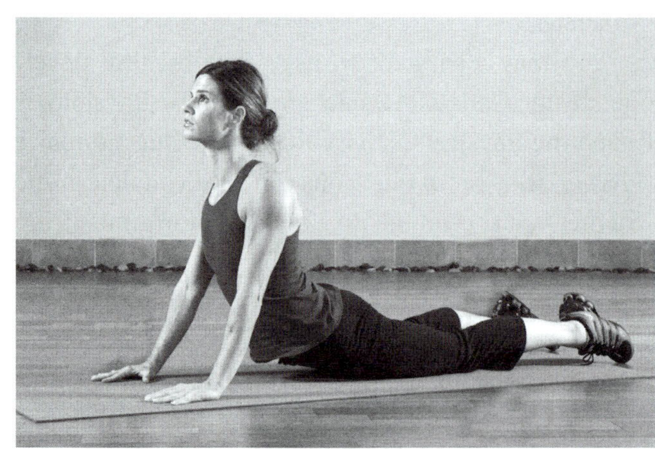

Although there isn't much scientific evidence favoring a cool-down following a light to moderate workout, the end of your session is an excellent time to stretch since your muscles are well warmed up.

- **Respect the weather.** When humidity is high or the thermometer is expected to reach 80° F, exercise during cooler morning or evening hours or in an air-conditioned space. When exercising outside in cold weather, dress in layers, including gloves and hat. If you have asthma or other respiratory problems, plan to exercise indoors when air quality is especially unhealthy. Seasonal allergy sufferers benefit from moving indoors, too, when pollen counts are high or other allergens abound.
- **Stay hydrated.** Drink sufficient fluids throughout the day and while exercising, especially if it's hot or humid.

Five strength training safety tips

When doing strength training, including the workouts in this report, follow these tips to help prevent injury.

- **Use light weight or resistance only.** Strength is built by working a muscle against resistance. (Exercise programs that do this are called strength training, resistance training, or weight training programs.) The resistance can be supplied by a hand weight like a dumbbell; elastic resistance bands or tubing; a weight machine; or your own body weight, as push-ups neatly illustrate. All of the workouts in this report emphasize building up muscle strength very slowly. When an exercise calls for hand weights, use no more than 1 to 3 pounds. When using resistance bands and tubing, select light to medium resistance.
- **Focus on form.** Good form means aligning your body as described in exercise instructions and moving smoothly through an exercise (see "Posture and alignment," page 8). Holding your body in a specific position while consciously contracting and releasing certain muscles allows you to isolate a muscle group. Poor form can slow gains and trigger injuries.
- **Tempo, tempo.** Work evenly at the tempo specified in each exercise. Control is very important. Counting off the tempo aloud helps you stay in control, which enhances gains and helps you avoid injuries. It also ensures that you're breathing, rather than holding your breath.
- **Breathe.** Blood pressure rises if you hold your breath during resistance exercises. Exhale as you work against gravity by lifting, pushing, or pulling; inhale as you release. During warm-ups and stretches, breathe comfortably.
- **Give muscles time off.** Strength training causes tiny tears in muscle tissue. Muscles grow stronger as the tears knit up. Allow at least 48 hours between strength training sessions on a particular group of muscles to allow them to recover.

Hip bone connected to the thighbone

The old song "Dry Bones" had it right. The toe bone is connected to the foot bone, and the foot bone is connected to the ankle bone, and so on up the long, linked chain of bones that make up a complete skeleton. The result: misalignment in one area tends to cause problems elsewhere in the body.

For example, injuring your left ankle completely alters your gait. To take the weight off the painful foot, you move more quickly than usual on your left side, lurching forward repeatedly onto your right leg. This potent combination of force and misalignment can trigger bursitis and pain in your right hip. Thus, new problems may zigzag up the body, making you vulnerable to further injuries, particularly if muscles supporting other joints are weak. If your body stages a general slowdown in response to all the new discomforts, other muscles eventually become deconditioned, too.

Take steps to minimize misalignments, when possible. Be aware of pain and restrictions in range of motion as you increase your physical activity. Pause occasionally to take stock of your body position and actively practice good posture. Wear supportive shoes (and orthotics to align your feet properly if your doctor feels you need them). Choose bags that distribute weight evenly, such as backpacks.

Four stretching safety tips

Using proper technique for stretching can protect your muscles and joints.

- **Warm up first.** Much like taffy, muscles stretch more easily when warm. Doing the warm-ups for each workout or taking a warm shower or bath will do the trick. Muscles also warm up from exercise, so the end of your workout is a great time to improve flexibility.
- **Feel no pain.** Stretch only to the point of mild tension, never to the point of pain. If a stretch hurts, stop immediately! Reset your position carefully and

try again. With time and practice, your flexibility will improve. (If you have arthritis, however, some degree of discomfort is to be expected. Try the two-hour rule: if discomfort following stretches lasts longer than two hours, or is more severe than your usual pain, step your routine down by holding stretches for less time or going less deeply into a stretch.)

- **Don't bounce.** It's tempting to move deeper into a stretch by bouncing. However, that can injure muscles if the movements are not carefully controlled. Sudden movements trigger the so-called stretch reflex, which causes a lengthening muscle to shorten. Instead, move slowly. If you try to quickly touch your toes, you may not be able to do it, but if you reach toward your toes as far as if comfortable, then hang for 15 to 30 seconds, your muscles will slowly lengthen, enabling you to get closer to your target.
- **Practice often.** You'll see the best gains if you stretch frequently—several times a day on as many days of the week as possible.

Posture and alignment

Posture counts when you're exercising. Aligning your body properly is the key to good form, which results in greater gains and fewer injuries (see "Hip bone connected to the thighbone," page 7). Few people have perfect posture, so we recommend quick posture checks before and during each exercise. If possible, look in a mirror as you do each exercise.

Do quick posture checks before and during each exercise.

When an exercise in our workouts calls for you to stand up straight, that means

- chin parallel to the floor
- both shoulders even (roll them up, back, and down to help achieve this)
- both arms at your sides with elbows straight and even
- abdominal muscles pulled in
- both hips even
- both knees even and pointing straight ahead
- both feet pointing straight ahead
- body weight distributed evenly on both feet.

Whether you're standing or seated, neutral posture requires you to keep your chin parallel to the floor; your shoulders, hips, and knees at even heights; and your knees and feet pointing straight ahead. A neutral spine takes into account the slight natural curves of the spine—don't flex it or arch it to overemphasize the curve of the lower back. A neutral wrist is firm and straight, not bent upward or downward. And neutral alignment means keeping your body in a straight line from head to toe except for the slight natural curves of the spine.

Equipment: Choosing the right stuff

We designed our workouts for home or gym. Look at the start of each workout description to see what equipment you'll need; each workout uses some, not all, of the equipment listed below. When equipment is listed as optional, you'll need it if you choose to do a harder or easier variation of certain exercises. Below are some buying tips for each of the items mentioned in our workouts.

Ankle weights. These are used to increase resistance in the harder variations of certain exercises. Choose padded, adjustable ankle weights with 1-pound bars so you can vary the weight as needed.

Chair. Choose a sturdy chair that won't tip over easily. A plain wooden dining chair without arms or heavy padding works well.

Hand weights. Our joint workouts use very light weights of 1 to 3 pounds, or occasionally 3 to 5 pounds. D-shaped weights and padded weights are easier to hold. Kits that let you screw weights onto a central bar save storage space.

Hand towel. A small hand towel tucked under your elbow anchors your upper arm during a few exercises. This helps isolate the muscles that the exercise is designed to strengthen. Any hand towel will do.

Mat. Choose a well-padded, nonslip mat for floor exercises. Yoga mats are readily available. A thick carpet or towels will do in a pinch.

Resistance bands. These wide, stretchy strips are available in several levels of resistance, designated by different colors and ranging from very light to very heavy. Resistance bands are often used for rehabilitation exercises after injuries or surgery. The strips can be knotted into a loop when an exercise requires this (see "Point and flex," page 23), or tied securely around a column, banister, or doorknob. Choose light- to medium-resistance bands in 6-foot lengths (or cut rolls of bands to this length yourself).

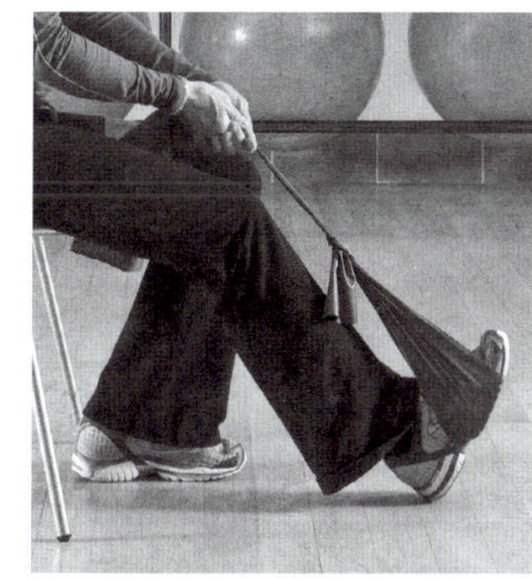

Before each use, make sure your resistance band has no nicks or cuts that will cause it to break. For safety, replace resistance bands often.

Resistance tubing. Look for tubing in several levels of resistance and with padded handles on the ends. Different colors designate varying amounts of resistance from very light to very heavy. For these workouts, choose light to medium resistance. Also look for a brand with a door attachment, which allows you to anchor the tubing in place when doing certain exercises.

Rubber ball. Choose a ball you can comfortably fit in your hand. The squishier the ball, the easier the workout, so select a firmer rubber ball when you're ready for more of a challenge.

Shoes. Choosing the right shoe for the task—running, walking, tennis, golf—is important. Running or walking shoes lose cushioning and support over time, so be sure to replace them regularly. Some experts suggest buying new ones every 350 to 550 miles.

Stability ball. Stability balls come in several sizes (55 cm, 65 cm, and 75 cm are most common, but smaller and larger balls are available). To select a ball, check the package for a size chart based on your height. When you sit on a ball, your hips and knees should both be at 90-degree angles. Select a durable, high-quality ball.

Yoga strap. This is a nonelastic cotton or nylon strap of 6 feet or longer that helps you position your body properly while doing certain stretches. Choose a strap with a D-ring or buckle fastener on one end. This allows you to put a loop around a foot or leg and then grasp the other end of the strap.

Getting started

Often, the slide toward an increasingly sedentary life starts with painful joints, because discomfort curtails activities. Although a doctor may prescribe temporary rest after an injury or surgery, week after week of inactivity compromises your health and abilities. Our simple walking plan can help you turn around this unhealthy trend. If walking isn't possible, see "When walking hurts" on page 11 for alternative activities.

Walking: A simple cardio workout

Like all aerobic (cardio) activities, walking tunes up the heart and lungs while burning calories. Because it doesn't jar joints terribly or raise the heart rate to dangerous levels, it's safe for almost everyone. Our walking plan (below) ramps up slowly. Follow these tips to get the most from your walks:

Find safe places to walk. Quiet streets with sidewalks, park trails, athletic tracks at local schools, or indoor malls are safest. If you're looking for a flat surface, the latter two choices are best.

Buy a good pair of shoes. Look for thick, flexible soles that cushion your feet and elevate your heel a half to three-quarters of an inch above the sole. Choose shoes with "breathable" uppers, such as nylon mesh or leather.

Dress for comfort and safety. Since exercise warms your body, wear lighter clothes than you'd need if standing still. Dress in layers so you can peel off garments if you get hot. Wear a hat with a brim

A walking plan

Our walking plan (at right) is designed to safely boost your physical activity even if you are very sedentary. It's the minutes that count, not the miles. If you aren't in the habit of exercising, start at the beginning. If you're already exercising, start at the level that best matches your current routine and build from there. You may advance more slowly by repeating a level for an additional week. (If walking is too painful, see "When walking hurts," page 11.)

Or, if the plan is too easy, you may add walking time more quickly. Once you're in shape, feel free to change time and days while still aiming for at least 150 minutes of walking per week. Looking for still more of a challenge? Add distance or hills to improve endurance.

Remember:

- Begin your walk at a slower pace for several minutes to warm up.
- If you like, you can divide daily walking time into chunks of 5 to 10 minutes.
- A brisk (moderate) pace makes singing difficult, but you should be able to talk.
- After your walk is an excellent time to stretch warmed muscles.

Week	Sessions per week	Daily minutes of brisk walking	Total weekly minutes
Week 1	2	5	10
Week 2	3	5	15
Week 3	4	5	20
Week 4	5	5	25
Week 5	5	10	50
Week 6	5	20	100
Week 7	5	25	125
Week 8	5	30	150

One way to measure walking speed is to count steps per minute with a watch and pedometer. A moderate (brisk) walking speed is a safe goal for most people. Provided you're walking on level ground, you can use the following as general guidance to gauge your pace:

Slow = 80 steps per minute
Moderate (brisk) = 100 steps per minute
Fast = 120 steps per minute
Race walking = More than 120 steps per minute

Table 1: Real-life metabolic equivalents (METs)

METs	Sample activities	Approximate calories used per hour by a 155-pound person
1	Sitting, reading, desk work, watching TV	70
1.1–2.5	Office work, city driving, standing in line	175
2.6–4.4	Housework, normal walking, light gardening, bowling, slow dancing, tai chi, yoga, brisk walking	175–310
4.5–5.9	Baseball, calisthenics, downhill skiing, cycling, swimming, golfing (carrying clubs)	315–415
6–8.4	Jogging, competitive sports, singles tennis	420–590
8.5 or more	Sprinting, jogging uphill, fast running, unusually heavy work	595+

and sunblock when needed. Light-colored clothes and reflective strips, a reflective vest, or a lightweight flashing light can help drivers notice you.

Do a warm-up. Walk at a slower pace for several minutes as you start out.

Practice good technique. Try not to shuffle, but to use good form. For example:

- Walk at a steady, moderate-intensity pace. Slow down if you're too breathless to carry on a conversation.
- Keep your head up and back straight. Lift your chest and shoulders. Gently contract your stomach muscles.
- Keeping toes pointed straight ahead, land on your heel, then roll forward onto the ball of your foot and push off from your toes. Walking flat-footed or only on the ball of your foot may lead to soreness and fatigue. Take long, easy strides, letting your arms swing loosely at your sides.
- If you want to boost your speed, bend your elbows at a 90-degree angle and swing your hands from waist to chest height. Take quicker steps, not longer ones.
- When walking faster or going up hills, lean forward slightly.

Stretch after walking. Stretching when your muscles are warm improves your range of motion.

When walking hurts

Strengthening muscles that support weak hip, knee, or ankle joints and working on flexibility can help you return to walking comfortably. But if our walking plan is too painful for you right now, try some of these lower-impact options for aerobic activity:

- elliptical trainer
- hand-crank bike
- kayaking simulator
- recumbent or upright stationary bike
- rowing machine
- recumbent or upright stepper
- swimming
- water aerobics
- water walking.

By working large muscles and bumping up your heart rate and breathing to circulate oxygen more throughout your body, all of these choices enhance cardiovascular fitness as well as walking does, while going easy on the joints. Some types of equipment—like elliptical trainers, kayaking simulators, and recumbent stationary bikes—are available at gyms and exercise rehabilitation centers.

Other excellent forms of low-impact exercise include

- qigong
- tai chi
- yoga.

Though these three types of exercise are not considered aerobic, they strengthen muscles and increase flexibility. New evidence indicates that yoga has some cardiovascular benefits as well.

Why weight matters for joint pain

Being overweight raises your risk for developing osteoarthritis in a weight-bearing joint like the knee. (Some research indicates that it may even contribute to arthritis in non-weight-bearing joints like those in the hand, since inflammatory factors related to weight might exacerbate this condition.) Simply walking across level ground puts up to one-and-a-half times your body weight on your knees. That means a 200-pound man will deliver 300 pounds of pressure to his knee with each step. Off level ground, the news is worse: each knee bears two to three times your body weight when you go up and down stairs, and four to five times your body weight when you squat to tie a shoelace or pick up an item you dropped.

Fortunately, strengthening your thigh muscles changes the equation, and so does losing weight. Each pound you lose reduces knee pressure in every step you take. One study found that the risk of developing osteoarthritis dropped 50% with each 11-pound weight loss among younger obese women. If older men lost enough weight to shift from an obese classification to just overweight—that is, from a body mass index (BMI) of 30 or higher down to one that fell between 25 and 29.9—the researchers estimated knee osteoarthritis would decrease by a fifth. For older women, that shift would cut knee osteoarthritis by a third.

To find your BMI, see Table 2 (below).

The best tactics for losing weight

Aerobic activity, such as walking, is best for aiding in weight loss and helping you maintain a healthy weight. But by itself, stepping up activity is rarely enough to help you lose weight (see "Why it's tough to lose weight with activity alone," page 13). You need to be aware of

Table 2: Normal, overweight, or obese?

The body mass index (BMI) is an index of weight by height. The definitions of normal, overweight, and obese were established after researchers examined the BMIs of millions of people and correlated them with rates of illness and death. These studies identified the normal BMI range as that associated with the lowest rates of illness and death. Obesity has been further subdivided into three classes. People may be candidates for weight-loss surgery if they have class III obesity, or if they have class II obesity and diabetes or another serious, weight-related medical condition.

HEIGHT	BODY WEIGHT IN POUNDS				
4′10″	89–119	120–143	144–167	168–191	192+
4′11″	92–124	125–148	149–173	174–198	199+
5′0″	95–128	129–153	154–179	179–204	205+
5′1″	98–132	133–158	159–185	186–211	212+
5′2″	101–136	137–164	165–191	192–218	219+
5′3″	105–141	142–169	170–197	198–225	226+
5′4″	108–145	146–174	175–204	205–232	233+
5′5″	111–150	151–180	181–210	211–240	241+
5′6″	115–155	156–186	187–216	217–247	248+
5′7″	118–159	160–191	192–223	224–255	256+
5′8″	122–164	165–197	198–230	231–262	263+
5′9″	126–169	170–203	204–236	237–270	271+
5′10″	129–174	175–209	210–243	244–278	279+
5′11″	133–179	180–215	216–250	251–286	287+
6′0″	137–184	185–221	222–258	259–294	295+
6′1″	140–189	190–227	228–265	266–302	303+
6′2″	145–194	195–233	234–272	273–311	312+
6′3″	149–200	201–240	241–279	279–319	320+
6′4″	153–205	206–246	247–287	288–328	329+
BMI	**18.5–24.9** NORMAL	**25–29.9** OVERWEIGHT	**30–34.9** CLASS I OBESITY	**35–39.9** CLASS II OBESITY	**40+** CLASS III OBESITY

Why it's tough to lose weight with activity alone

You would expect pounds ought to peel off easily as your activity level rises. Alas, it rarely works this way. There are several reasons for this seeming contradiction.

You don't burn as many calories as you think. As you're lifting weights at the gym or striding around the block at a brisk clip, it's easy to imagine how many calories you're incinerating. The actual amount can be surprisingly low. Walking or jogging uses up roughly 100 calories per mile (though the precise amount varies with your weight and pace, with a heavier person and faster pace burning more). Since there are 3,500 calories to a pound of fat, that means you'd need to walk 35 miles to lose 1 pound—assuming your levels of food intake and other physical activity remain the same.

Virtue is rarely its own reward. Ever treat yourself to a cookie or an extra dollop of dinner on a day when you walked or worked out? It's a common impulse that undermines your efforts. However much you burn through exercise, it's incredibly easy to replace that amount with a post-workout snack: 20 minutes of brisk walking burns 69 calories for a 120-pound person; 86 calories for a 150-pound person; and 103 calories for a 180-pound person. But a small cookie can cost you 50 to 60 calories, a serving of chips tallies 150 calories, and a half cup of ice cream can be 140 calories (and many of us scoop more than that into our bowls). Healthier rewards range from appreciating the effects of exercise—feeling more energetic, calmer, or stronger, for example—to planning a night out or promising yourself new exercise gear or new music if you stick with your program.

Your metabolic rate slows with weight loss. Even if you loll around in bed all day, you burn off a certain number of calories. This number is known as your basal metabolic rate (BMR), and it reflects the amount of energy your body needs to carry out basic functions, such as breathing, making the heart beat, and generating heat. Any exercise or physical activity you get burns off additional calories. However, when you lose weight, your BMR decreases, so you're not burning as many calories any more through these basic functions. To maintain weight loss, you need to lower your calorie intake to match your body's needs. If you're curious about how many calories you need to maintain your current weight (or to lose weight), run your vital stats through an online calculator for basal metabolic rate and calories burned for different types of activities. For some examples of calories burned through normal activity, see Table 1, page 11.

calories, too. Every pound you'd like to shed represents roughly 3,500 calories. So, if you're hoping to lose half a pound to 1 pound a week, you need to knock off 250 to 500 calories a day. Vaporizing half through exercising and half by cutting calories from your diet is a good mix. Aiming at the lower number—125 calories shed through exercise and 125 calories shaved off your diet—can help ensure success.

It's wise to keep in mind that the math works in the other direction, too: if you don't burn a single calorie through exercise and you add 250 calories a day through more nibbling, you'd rack up an extra 26 pounds a year. Indulging in just an extra 100 calories a day without burning them off packs on 10 pounds a year. Over time, daily indulgences like a scoop or two of ice cream, an energy bar, or a raid on the cookie or candy jar can tip the scales against you.

What sort of diet is best? Try to stick with a diet that emphasizes healthy choices: lots of fruits, vegetables, and whole grains; fish, lean poultry, beans, and legumes as protein sources; healthful oils; and a sprinkling of nuts.

Dig deep for motivation

Need more motivation to make a start or stick to it? Welcome to the club. Often, the hardest part of a workout is mustering the drive to get up and go. While exercise is great medicine, it only works if you do it regularly. Here are a few tips:

Find the time. Get up half an hour earlier each day for a morning workout. If big blocks of time aren't falling into your lap, break it up. Try 10-minute walks, or half a workout in the morning and half in the evening. Skip several half-hour TV shows a week—or work out while watching. Many gyms have TV monitors next to exercise machines. You can also buy a mini-cycle to pedal in place while watching TV at home.

Build active moments into your day. Start small and build up by choosing among options like these: Take stairs, not elevators. When commuting, get off the bus or subway a stop or two ahead, or park farther away from your workplace. While on the phone, try a few stretches, pace, or do simple exercises like lunges, squats, and heel raises.

Bike or walk to work, if possible. When running errands within a reasonable radius, park your car in

My monthly log: Planning your workouts and walking program

WEEK	MONDAY	TUESDAY	WEDNESDAY
Example	*Ankles: Full workout 7:30–8:00 p.m. Walking 12:30–12:50 p.m.*	*Walking 12:30–12:50 p.m.*	*Ankles: Full workout 7:30–8:00 p.m.*
1			
2			
3			
4			
5			

one spot and walk to different shops. Replace your desk and desk chair with a standing desk or treadmill desk. Try substituting a stability ball for your desk chair for a few hours a day. Rake leaves and shovel snow instead of using a leaf blower or snowblower.

Find a workout buddy. Workouts with a friend are more fun, plus you're less likely to cancel on the spur of the moment.

Brainstorm solutions. Understanding likely bumps in the road and planning solutions can help keep you on track.

- **Need the okay to start exercising?** Call your doctor today. It may help to fax or send a copy of the workout and walking plan, then follow up with a phone call to discuss it.
- **Bugged by bad weather or early darkness?** Buy equipment necessary for exercising at home, join a gym, try a class in your community, or walk the mall or an indoor athletic track at a local school.
- **Feeling sick?** Take time off to recover, then start at an easier-than-usual pace and work back up.
- **Bored?** Join a class, change up your exercise routine, or find a workout buddy.
- **Unmotivated?** Remind yourself of your goals, plan small rewards, ask a friend to check up on you, or consider working out with a personal trainer.
- **Not sure what to do?** Join a class with an instructor who can teach you the movements, or make an appointment with a personal trainer for one-on-one instruction. Paying for expertise and having an appointment can be powerful motivators.

Now it's your turn. Complete the planning worksheet on page 16, brainstorming solutions as you go. Then fill out the monthly log below.

THURSDAY	FRIDAY	SATURDAY	SUNDAY
Walking *12:30–12:50 p.m.*	*Walking* *12:30–12:50 p.m.*	*Walking* *12:30–12:50 p.m.*	

Planning worksheet

Filling in this worksheet will help you set goals and jump hurdles. Start by listing what you stand to gain. This could be the extra push you need to stay on track. Also note how active you are now, so you'll know if you're getting sufficient exercise to stay healthy and independent (see "How much exercise should you aim for?" on page 3).

Make a copy of this worksheet. Write down your answers, then fill in the monthly log. Tack it up on your refrigerator or another spot where you'll see it every day. Share your goals with family and friends, so that they can encourage you, too.

1. What will I gain?

Is your shoulder keeping you away from tennis or making it hard to lift a child, grandchild, or bag of groceries? Has your knee put the kibosh on walking, hikes, running, or just climbing stairs comfortably? Think about what you're missing out on, what you need to be able to do, and what you might enjoy trying.

My first goal is to

- ❑ strengthen my ankles so I can

  ____

- ❑ strengthen my knees so I can

  ____

- ❑ strengthen my shoulders so I can

  ____

- ❑ strengthen my hips so I can

  ____

- ❑ strengthen my wrists and elbows so I can

  ____

My additional goals are to

- ❑ enhance my overall health
- ❑ tone my muscles
- ❑ extend my endurance
- ❑ improve my balance
- ❑ lose __________ pounds in the next __________ weeks for the benefit of my knees and all-around health. (Work toward an initial goal of losing 5% to 10% of your weight by losing half a pound to 1 pound a week. If you weigh 200 pounds, that's 10 to 20 pounds.)

I'd like to

- ❑ do the ankle workout
- ❑ do the knee workout
- ❑ do the hip workout
- ❑ do the shoulder workout
- ❑ do the wrist and elbow workout
- ❑ add the walking program or another cardio workout to enhance my overall health and improve my endurance.

2. How can I make it over the hurdles?

What might keep you from exercising regularly? When you run into hurdles—boredom, time crunches, and other common setbacks—reminding yourself of the pledges below can help you make it over them. It pays to think ahead about what might derail you, then brainstorm solutions that will help you stick with your plan. Here are some solutions for common problems.

- ❑ I will stay excited by rotating activities and trying out new sports, interactive computer games, fitness tracking devices, dancing, or other enjoyable activities.
- ❑ I will plan ahead for short winter days and tough weather conditions (too hot, too cold, too icy, too rainy, too humid) by finding indoor spaces for my workouts, such as a gym, fitness studio, community center, mall, or my home.
- ❑ If I find it hard to exercise at the end of a long day, I'll choose times of day when I feel more energetic.
- ❑ I will make small promises I can keep, allowing me to celebrate successes and make slow, steady gains.
- ❑ I will make a game out of finding as many ways as possible to slip exercise into my day through simple steps like taking the stairs, walking the dog, parking in one spot to run several errands, marching or jogging in place during TV commercials, or fitting in a few stretches or exercises before meals, during breaks, or even while on the phone.
- ❑ I will invite friends, family, or co-workers to join me for walks, sports, and interactive games—and possibly even match me in friendly competition (biggest exerciser, anyone?).

What else might help me stick to my plan?

____

____

3. My plan

Make copies of the monthly log on pages 14 and 15, then jot down the title of the workout you'll do, penciling in the time slot and day you've chosen. Remember the advice to start slow and build gradually. Pencil in your walking program, too, by adding time and days from "A walking plan" on page 10. Then check off every workout you complete. Asking a friend to hold you accountable—or striking a similar bargain with your doctor—may encourage you to exercise. If so, copy the completed log and send it to your friend or doctor at the end of each month.

Using the workouts

This chapter explains terms used in the workouts and answers six common questions.

What information is in each exercise?

When you turn to the workout you've chosen—for instance, shoulders or knees—you'll find each exercise has certain specific information and instructions. Following are definitions of the terms we've used.

Starting position. This describes how to position your body before starting the exercise.

Movement. Here you'll find out how to perform the exercise correctly.

Repetitions (or reps). Each time you complete the full movement, that's a rep. It's fine if you can't do all the reps at first. Focus on quality—good form comes first—rather than quantity. Gradually increase reps as you improve.

Sets. One set is a specific number of repetitions. In our workouts, 10 reps typically add up to a single set. Usually, we suggest doing one to three sets.

Intensity. Intensity measures how hard you work during an exercise. Pay attention to objective physiological cues like breathing, talking, and sweating, or you can measure intensity subjectively through perceived exertion (see Table 3, at right).

Tempo. This provides the count for the key movements in an exercise. Here's how the 3-1-3 tempo works in "Wall push-up with stability ball" (see page 39): Slowly count to 3 while bending your elbows to lower your upper body toward the wall. Pause for one second. Then count to 3 again as you return to the starting position. To avoid hurrying, it helps to count while watching or listening to seconds tick by on a clock. When you can no longer maintain the recommended tempo, stop that exercise even if you haven't finished all of the reps.

Hold. Hold tells you the number of seconds to pause while holding a pose during an exercise. You'll see this in stretches, which are held 10 to 30 seconds. While starting out at 10 seconds is fine, gradually extending that until you can comfortably hold the stretch for 30 seconds will give you better results. So, too, will practicing flexibility exercises every day rather than just a few times a week.

Rest. Resting gives your muscles a chance to recharge, which helps you maintain good form. No rest is needed during warm-ups or after stretches unless otherwise specified.

Tips and techniques. We offer two or three pointers to help you maintain good form and make the greatest gains from the exercise.

Too hard? This section gives you an option for making the exercise easier.

Too easy? This section gives you an option for making the exercise more challenging.

Table 3: How hard am I working?

INTENSITY	IT FEELS...	YOU ARE...
Light	Easy	• Breathing easily • Warming up, but not yet sweating • Able to talk—or even sing an aria if you have the talent
Light to moderate	You're working, but not too hard	• Breathing easily • Sweating lightly • Still finding it easy to talk or sing
Moderate	You're working	• Breathing faster • Starting to sweat more • Able to talk, not able to sing
Moderate to high	You're really working	• Huffing and puffing • Sweating • Able to talk in short sentences, but concentrating more on exercise than conversation
High	You're working very hard, almost out of gas	• Breathing hard • Sweating hard • Finding talking difficult

Before you start the workouts: An important warning

Did you recently injure your ankle, knee, hip, wrist, elbow, or shoulder? Are you experiencing significant pain or discomfort in any of these joints? Have you had surgery on a joint? If so, it's vital to talk to your doctor before embarking on the workout directed at that particular joint.

Depending on the situation, you may receive the go-ahead or may need to rest and take other measures to heal properly first. In some instances, a doctor might want to modify certain exercises or may recommend working with a physical therapist.

If you think pain relief could help you exercise more comfortably, discuss the options with your doctor. Examples include the following:

- **Over-the-counter pain relievers.** Naproxen (Aleve), ibuprofen (Advil), or acetaminophen (Tylenol) help reduce pain. Check with your doctor about the safest choice for you. Take 30 to 45 minutes before you do a workout.
- **Warm showers.** Showering before exercise helps warm up muscles and joints.
- **Cold.** Apply an ice wrap to the sore joint for 20 minutes after exercise.
- **Braces.** When needed, a brace can help support muscles, distribute force, and limit movement. Talk to your doctor about whether a brace would be helpful, and, if so, which kind to choose.

Answers to six common questions

If you haven't been working out regularly, or even if you have, you may have some questions about getting started on the workouts in this report.

1 | Which workout should I do?

That depends on which joints are bothering you. If it's an ankle, turn to "Ankle workout" (see page 20); if it's your hips, turn to "Hip workout" (see page 32). What if it's both? It's safe to do both routines as long as the problems you're experiencing are described in the workout introductions. If you have more significant joint problems, or if you have any doubts, see your doctor before you start any workout!

Pair the workout or workouts you choose with the weekly walking program or another choice (see "When walking hurts," page 11) to get the cardio tune-up your body needs.

2 | What if I can't do all the reps or sets suggested?

Quality is much more important than quantity. While you want to challenge yourself, it's okay if you can't do all the recommended reps or sets at the start. Begin by trying to finish a single set of each exercise in the workout, then gradually work up to more as you progress. Within any set, do only as many reps as you can manage while following instructions, maintaining good form, and sticking to the specified tempo. If necessary, try lightening up the weight or resistance to make this possible.

3 | How much weight or resistance should I use?

It's wise to have a selection of light weights (1, 2, and 3 pounds) and resistance tubing or bands (light through medium resistance).

Select the highest weight or level of resistance that allows you to accomplish all of the following:

- maintain good form throughout the exercise
- stick to the specified tempo
- complete the suggested number of reps and sets
- achieve a full and pain-free range of motion.

Wait until you find it easy to meet all four requirements before you increase the weight or resistance for a particular exercise. If it's difficult to meet any of the four, decrease the weight or resistance.

As you try the exercises, you'll find some muscle groups are stronger than other groups. Thus, you'll need to vary the amount of weight or resistance used in the course of your workout.

4 | How often should I do the exercises in a workout?

A full workout incorporates warm-ups, muscle strengthening exercises, and stretches. We recommend doing full workouts two to three times a week. Strenuous exercise like strength training causes tiny tears in muscle tissue. The muscles grow stronger as the tears knit up. Always allow at least 48 hours between strength training sessions to give the muscles time to recover. Warm-ups and stretches can be done more often—even daily—to enhance flexibility.

5 | When will I be ready to move on from a joint workout?

As long as you benefit from your workout, you may decide to stick with it. If you're itching to progress, though, you have several choices. When you can meet the four requirements described in question 3, do the following:

- Try the variation listed under the "Too easy?" heading for each exercise.
- Add weight or bump up resistance.
- Shift to a mainstream exercise program, preferably under the guidance of a fitness professional who can help you do this safely.

6 | How will I know I'm improving?

You can measure improvement in many ways. Before you launch your workouts, start by taking note of some basic information:

A. During a week, how often do you accumulate at least 30 minutes of moderate physical activity a day?

- **0–2 days:** To get started, see "A walking plan" on page 10 and focus on slow, steady gains.
- **3–4 days:** Great effort! If your time isn't adding up to 150 minutes or more weekly, however, try to shoehorn in brisk walks and similar activities on another day or two (see "When walking hurts" on page 11 if you're looking for other activities to try). Ten-minute chunks of activity are fine.
- **5+ days:** You've reached (or exceeded) your goal! Keep it up.

Ultimately, a healthy goal is achieving 150 minutes or more per week. It's perfectly fine to work up to that gradually. And remember, any activity is always better than none.

B. List three to five activities that are becoming more difficult to manage because of joint problems—for example, a daily activity like climbing the stairs, a household task like reaching overhead to take a package off a high shelf, or a sport you enjoy.

1. ______________________________
2. ______________________________
3. ______________________________
4. ______________________________
5. ______________________________

Six weeks after starting your workouts, take a moment to reassess the physical activity vital signs that you wrote down. Notice any improvements? Are you totting up more weekly minutes of activity or becoming active more days a week? Are the activities you listed becoming easier? If you're not quite there yet, applaud the strides you've made so far and keep trying.

Ankle workout

Your ankles must bear the full weight of your body, yet stay nimble and flexible. Every step, every jump, every dance move puts the ankle through a surprising range of motion. Even when you stand quietly, hips and knees at rest, the ankles are constantly moving and making minute adjustments to help you stay balanced.

Below you'll find brief descriptions of ankle anatomy and the joint problems that our ankle workout helps ease. The workout itself combines warm-ups, strength exercises to rebuild muscles that help protect your ankles, and stretches to improve ankle flexibility.

Ankles 101

People often take their ankles for granted, but these joints are actually quite complex (see Figure 1, at right). The large bone in the lower leg is the shin bone (tibia). It connects to the central ankle bone (talus). Bracketed by two bony bumps (each called a malleolus) on either side of the ankle, the talus acts as a hinge that allows you to point and flex your foot. Two other joints on the talus permit sideways movements. The shin bone bears all the weight; a second, smaller bone in the lower leg (fibula) ends alongside the talus. The heel bone (calcaneus) lies below the talus, cupping it. Two ligaments link the inner malleolus to the ankle bones. Three more ligaments bind the outer malleolus to the talus and calcaneus. Two large calf muscles, the gastrocnemius and soleus, are attached to the back of the foot by the strong, thick cord of the Achilles' tendon. A muscle at the front of the shin (tibialis anterior) lifts the front of the foot, and the gastrocnemius lifts the heel.

What this workout helps

Chronic ankle sprains. An ankle sprain, an injury so common the American Academy of Orthopaedic Surgeons estimates it happens 25,000 times a day, occurs when you roll your foot inward or outward, or turn or twist an ankle. That stretches, or even tears, the binding ligaments that keep the bones and joints properly positioned. Depending on the force applied as you land, the sprain can be mild, moderate, or severe. Repeated sprains make the ligaments lax, making additional sprains more likely. While sports involving running, jumping, or sudden stops and turns sometimes play a role in sprains, they may also occur simply when you walk on uneven ground or lose your balance.

Weak ankles. Weak muscles supporting the ankle affect balance and increase your vulnerability to injuries like sprains and falls.

Poor balance. Nerves in muscles and joints work with the vestibular system in your inner ear to constantly relay information about body movements and positioning. Called proprioception, this

Figure 1: Anatomy of the ankle

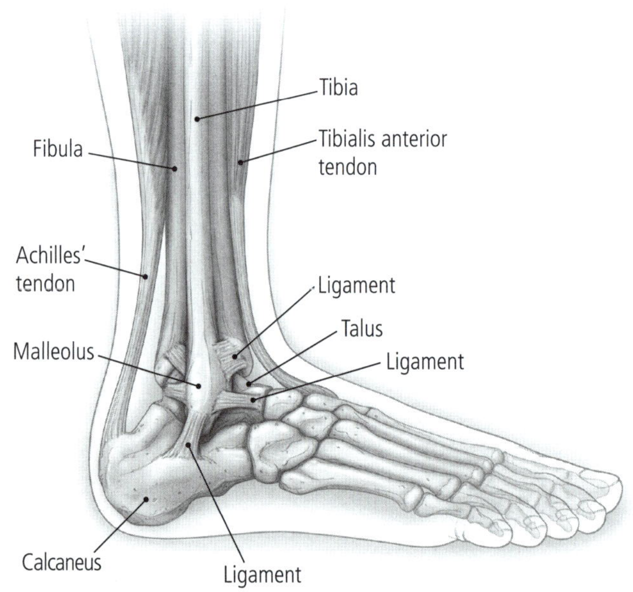

While you are standing, your ankle bears the full weight of your body and helps you stay balanced. The central ankle bone is the talus. The joint at this bone allows you to point and flex your foot while two other joints on the talus permit sideways movement.

sense operates independently of sight. By telling you where your ankle is in space, for example—stepping on a stair tread, perhaps, or recovering from a step onto uneven pavement—it helps you keep your balance. Like muscle strength, proprioception responds to training.

Ankle exercises

This workout strengthens ankles by building up supporting muscles that keep you balanced whether you're standing still, walking over changing terrain, or enjoying activities like dancing where you're moving in many directions. It helps increase much-needed flexibility in your ankles with stretches to release tight tendons, ligaments, and muscles. Plus, it enhances proprioception—the sense that tells you where your ankle is in space and helps you keep your balance. Ultimately, all of this can help prevent or limit falls.

We recommend performing the full workout two to three times a week. Make sure you leave 48 hours between strength exercise sessions to allow muscles time to recover. Warm-ups and stretches can be done daily to further enhance flexibility.

Equipment: Mat, resistance bands, sturdy chair, 1- to 3-pound ankle weights (optional), 3- to 5-pound dumbbells (optional).

Note: For this workout, take a length of resistance band and create a loop at one end of it, knotting it securely. Before each use, make sure there are no nicks or cuts in the band that could cause it to break.

1 | Warming up: **Ankle pumps**

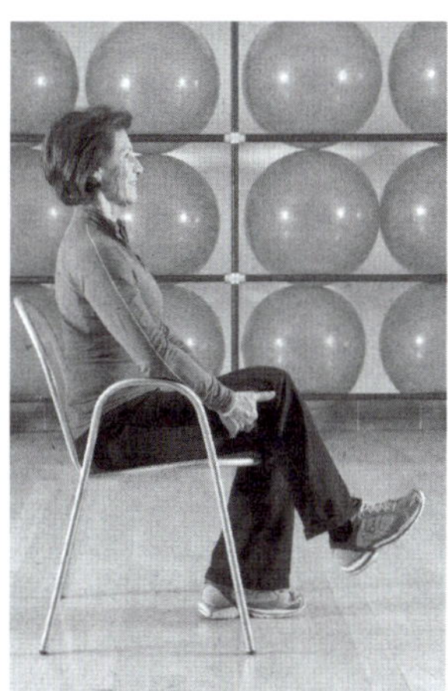

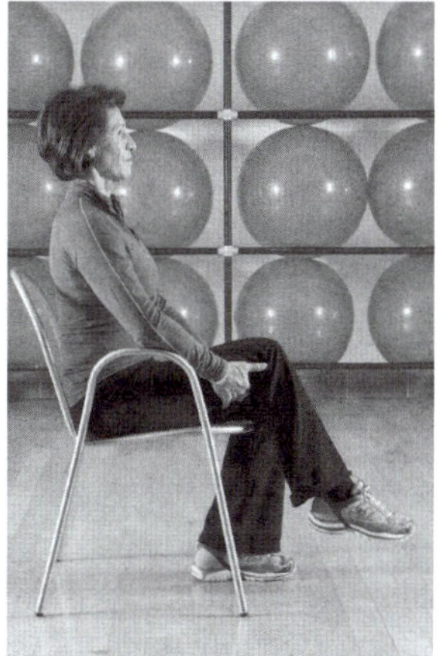

Reps: 10 per side
Sets: 1
Intensity: Light
Tempo: Slow and controlled
Rest: No rest needed

Starting position: Sit up straight in a chair with your feet flat on the floor. Lift your right foot a few inches off the floor.

Movement: Flex your foot to point your toes toward the ceiling. Then point your foot and toes toward the floor. Finish all reps, then repeat with your left leg. This completes one set.

Tips and techniques:

- Maintain neutral posture, with your shoulders down and back.
- Breathe comfortably.

Too hard? Make your movements smaller.
Too easy? Do two to three sets.

2 | Warming up: **Foot rotations**

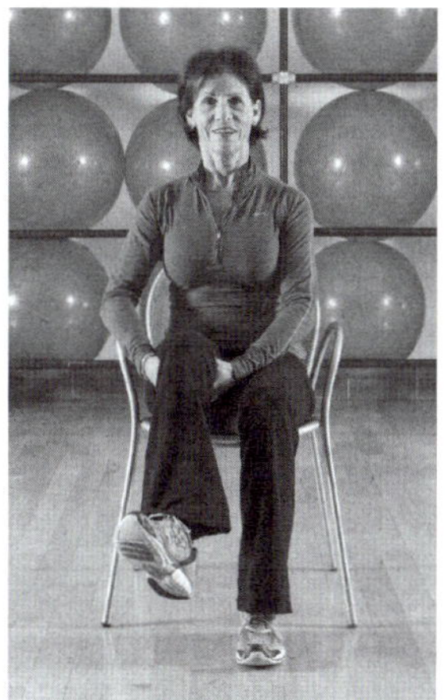

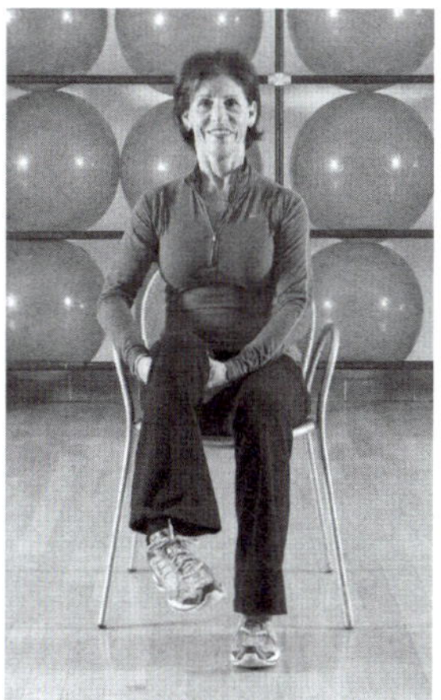

Reps: 10 in each direction per side
Sets: 1
Intensity: Light
Tempo: Slow and controlled
Rest: No rest needed

Starting position: Sit up straight in a chair.

Movement: Lift your right foot off the floor. Rotate your foot from the ankle in a circle going clockwise. Finish all reps, then repeat foot rotations going counterclockwise. Repeat circles in both directions with your left foot. This completes one set.

Tips and techniques:

- Maintain neutral posture, with your shoulders down and back.
- Breathe comfortably.

Too hard? Support your leg with both hands for assistance.
Too easy? Do two to three sets.

3 | Warming up: **Writing the alphabet**

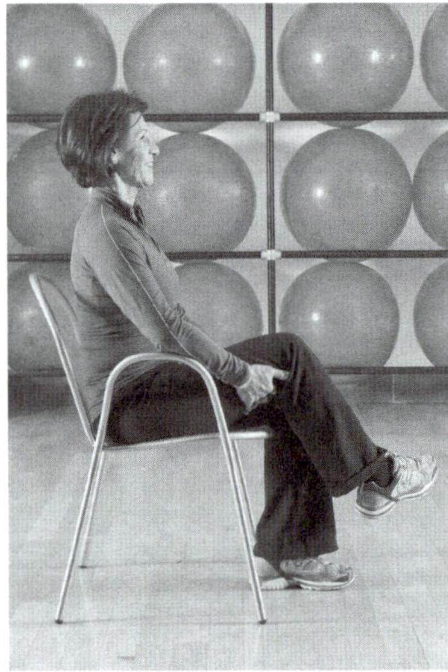

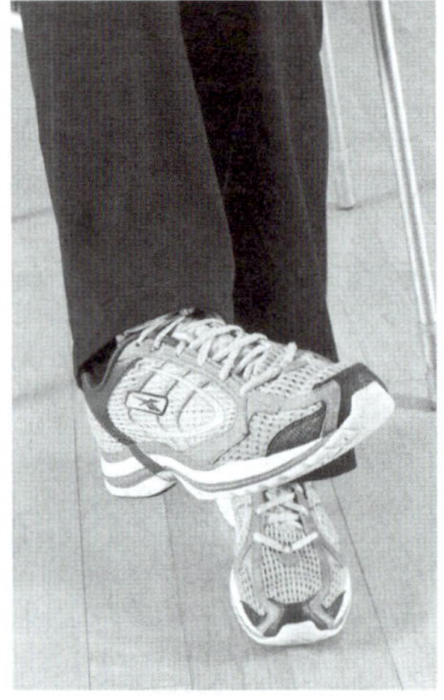

Reps: 1 per letter
Sets: 1
Intensity: Light
Tempo: Slow and controlled
Rest: No rest needed

Starting position: Sit up straight in a chair with your feet flat on the floor.

Movement: Lift your right foot a few inches off the floor and use your toes to write the alphabet in the air. The writing motions should come from the ankle. Repeat with the toes on your left foot. This completes one set.

Tips and techniques:

- Maintain neutral posture, with your shoulders down and back.
- Breathe comfortably.

Too hard? Support your leg with both hands for assistance.

Too easy? Do two to three sets.

4 | Strengthening: **Single leg stance**

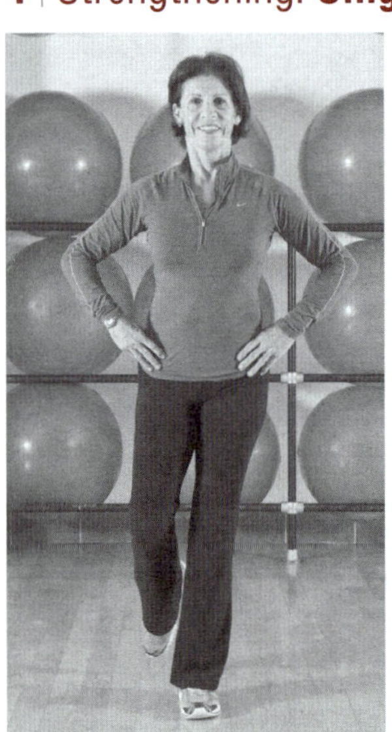

Reps: 1 per side
Sets: 1–3
Intensity: Moderate to hard
Hold: 60 seconds
Rest: 30–90 seconds between sets

Starting position: Stand up straight with your feet hip-width apart.

Movement: Lift your right foot a few inches off the floor, bending your knee slightly, and balancing on your left leg. Hold for 60 seconds, then lower your foot to the starting position. Repeat with your left leg lifted. This completes one set.

Tips and techniques:

- Maintain neutral posture, with your shoulders down and back.
- Tighten the muscles around your hips and buttocks for stability.
- Keep your abdominal muscles contracted.

Too hard? Hold on to a chair or counter for support, or hold for less than 60 seconds.

Too easy? Stand on a soft mat to make it more difficult to balance.

5 | Strengthening: **Heel raises**

Reps: 10
Sets: 1–3
Intensity: Light to moderate
Tempo: 3-1-3
Rest: 30–90 seconds between sets

Starting position: Stand up straight with your feet hip-width apart and your hands at your sides.

Movement: Slowly lift up on your toes so that your heels rise off the floor as high as possible. Pause, then slowly return to the starting position. This is one rep.

Tips and techniques:

- Maintain neutral posture, with your shoulders down and back.
- Stand evenly on your toes and heels before lifting and when returning to the starting position.
- Exhale as you lift.

Too hard? Hold on to a chair or counter for support.

Too easy? Hold weights (3 to 5 pounds) in your hands while doing the exercise.

6 | Strengthening: **Point and flex**

Reps: 10 of each step per side
Sets: 1–3
Intensity: Moderate
Tempo: 3-1-3
Rest: 30–90 seconds between sets

Starting position: Sit up straight in a chair with your feet flat on the floor. Extend your right leg with toes pointing toward the ceiling. Put the resistance band loop around the ball of your right foot like a sling. Hold the other end with both hands, keeping tension on it throughout the exercise.

Movement: This is a two-step exercise. **Step 1:** Slowly point your foot toward the floor, pause, then slowly return to the starting position. Finish all reps. **Step 2:** Place your right ankle on top of your left knee. Put the loop just below your right toes on top of the foot, keeping tension on this with your left hand. Slowly pull the toes of your right foot upward toward your right shin, pause, then slowly return to the Step 2 starting position. Finish all reps. Now repeat both steps with your left foot. This completes one set.

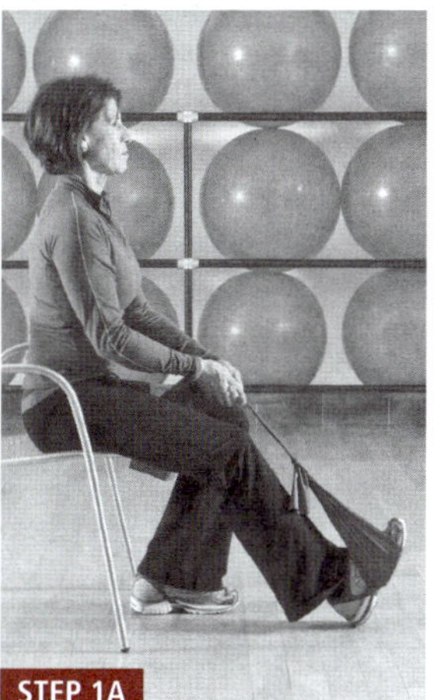
STEP 1A

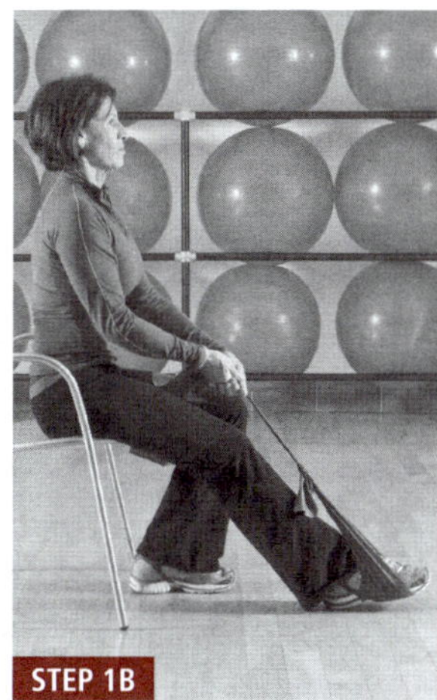
STEP 1B

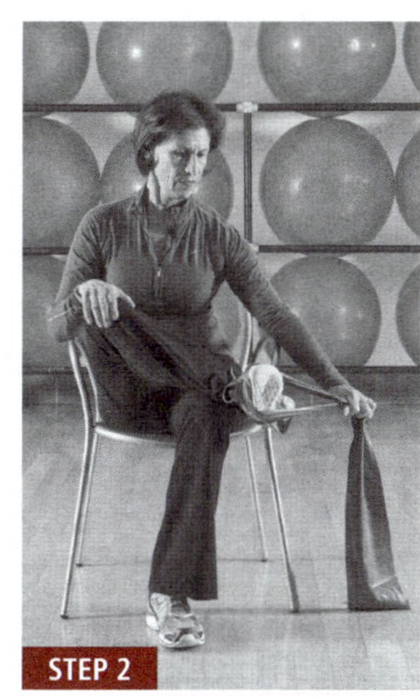
STEP 2

Tips and techniques:

- Keep tension on the band at all times to create resistance.
- Maintain neutral posture, with your shoulders down and back.
- Breathe comfortably.

Too hard? Use a lighter resistance band.
Too easy? Use a heavier resistance band.

7 | Strengthening: **Inversion and eversion**

Reps: 10 of each step per side
Sets: 1–3
Intensity: Moderate
Tempo: 3-1-3
Rest: 30–90 seconds between sets

Starting position: Sit on a mat with your legs extended. Bend your right knee and put the heel on the floor. Lift the toes toward the ceiling and place the loop of the resistance band around the ball of your right foot. Hold the band in your right hand, keeping tension on it.

Movement: This is a two-step exercise with a side-to-side movement. **Step 1:** Slowly turn your right foot inward. Pause, then return to center. Finish all reps. **Step 2:** Hold the band in your left hand, keeping tension on it. Slowly turn your right foot outward. Pause, then return to center. Finish all reps. Then repeat both steps with the loop on your left foot. This completes one set.

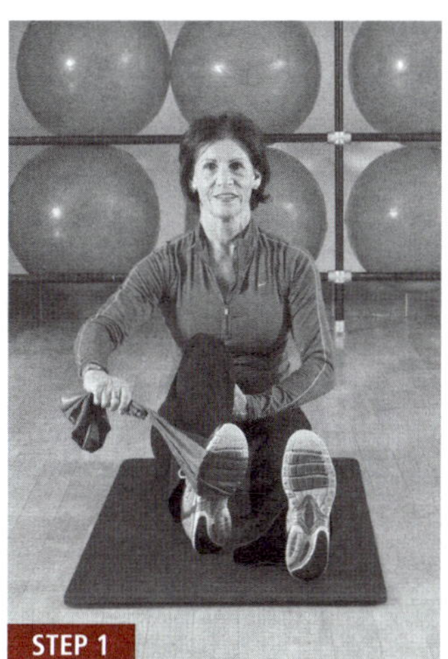
STEP 1

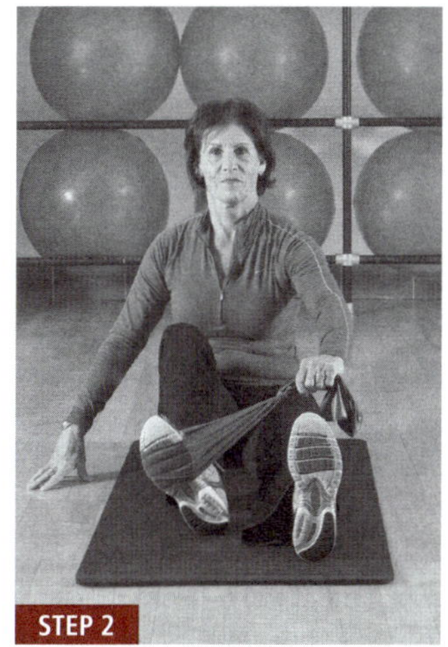
STEP 2

Tips and techniques:

- Keep tension on the band at all times to create resistance.
- Keep your heel on the floor throughout both steps.
- Maintain neutral posture, with your shoulders down and back.

Too hard? Sit against a wall and use a lighter resistance band.
Too easy? Use a heavier resistance band.

8 | Strengthening: **Toe taps**

Reps: 10 front, 10 side-to-side
Sets: 1–3
Intensity: Light to moderate
Tempo: 1-1
Rest: 30–90 seconds between sets

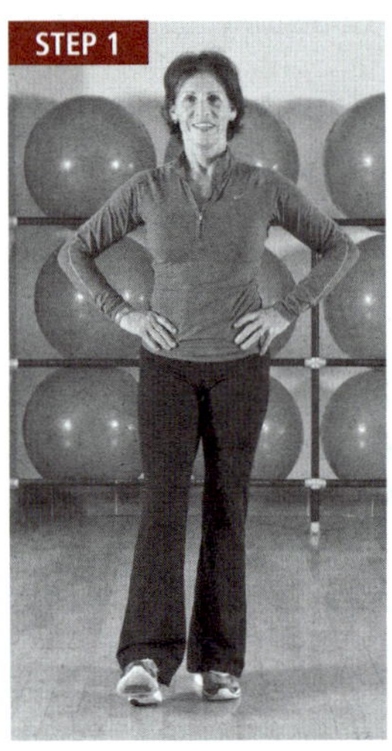
STEP 1

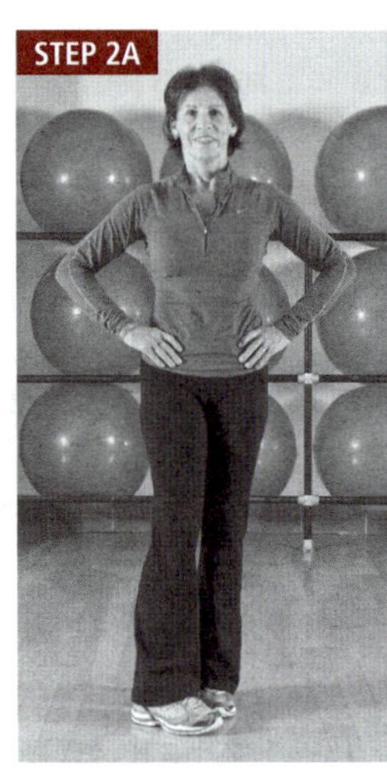
STEP 2A

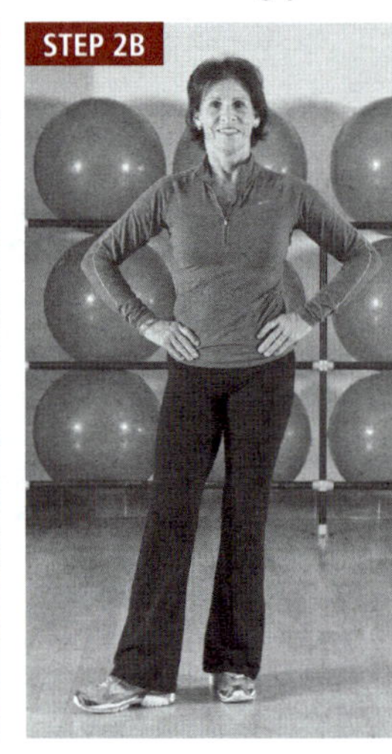
STEP 2B

Starting position: Stand up straight with your hands on your hips and your feet hip-width apart. Move your right foot forward so the right heel is in line with the toes of your left foot.

Movement: This is a two-step exercise. **Step 1:** While keeping your heel grounded on the floor, lift the toes of your right foot as high as you can and tap them on the floor 10 times. **Step 2:** Still keeping your heel grounded, lift up the toes of your right foot, then tap in and out (to the left and right) 10 times. Repeat both steps with your left foot. This completes one set.

Tips and techniques:

- Maintain neutral posture, with your shoulders down and back.
- Keep toe taps smooth and controlled.

Too hard? Perform the exercise while seated in a chair with both feet on the floor.

Too easy? Secure a 1- to 3-pound ankle weight around your foot behind the toes.

9 | Stretching: **Standing lower calf stretch**

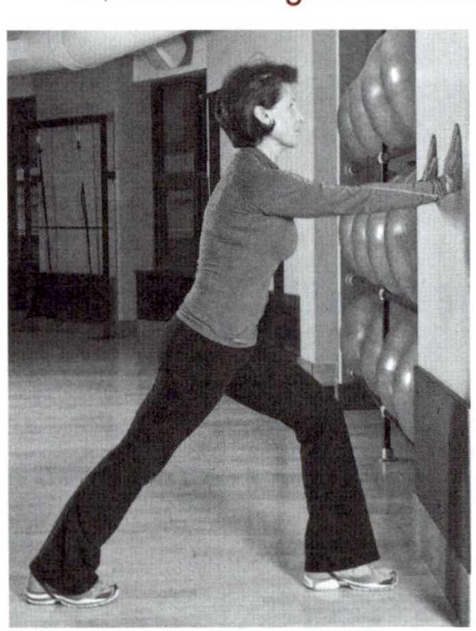

Reps: 3–4
Sets: 1
Intensity: Light
Hold: 10–30 seconds
Rest: No rest needed

Starting position: Stand up straight in front of a wall with your arms extended at shoulder height.

Movement: Place your hands on the wall. Extend your right leg straight back and press the heel toward the floor, feeling a stretch in the back of your right leg. Let your left leg bend as you do so to stabilize your body. Hold. Return to the starting position, then repeat with your left leg in back. This is one rep. Continue alternating feet until you finish all reps.

Tips and techniques:

- Stretch to the point of mild tension, not pain.
- Hold a full-body lean from the ankle as you stretch.
- Maintain neutral alignment, with your shoulders down and back.

Too hard? Hold the back of a chair and do not press as far into the stretch.

Too easy? Try to bend your back knee farther without lifting your heel off the floor. This increases the stretch.

10 | Stretching: **Standing soleus stretch**

Reps: 3–4 per side
Sets: 1
Intensity: Light
Hold: 10–30 seconds
Rest: No rest needed

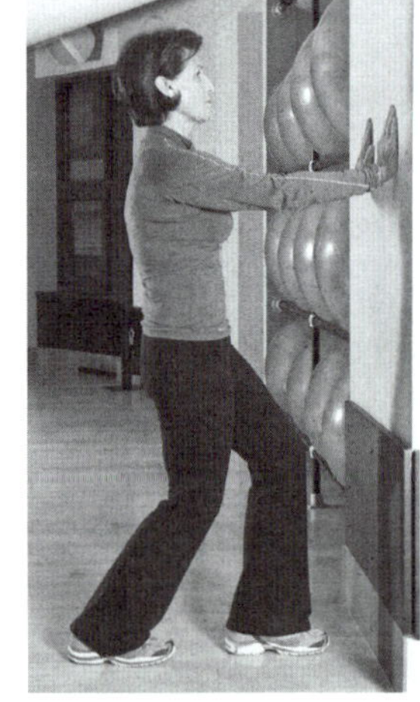

Starting position: Stand up straight in front of a wall with your arms extended at shoulder height.

Movement: Place your hands on the wall. Extend your right leg straight back and press the heel toward the floor. Let your left knee bend slightly as you do so, while keeping the heel grounded on the floor. Now bend your right knee as much as possible without lifting the heel off the floor, feeling a stretch in the calf of your right leg. Hold. Return to the starting position. Finish all reps, then repeat with your left foot. This completes one set.

Tips and techniques:

- Stretch to the point of mild tension, not pain.
- Maintain neutral posture, with your shoulders down and back.

Too hard? Hold the back of a chair and do not press as far into the stretch.

Too easy? Try to bend your back knee farther without lifting your heel off the floor. This increases the stretch.

11 | Stretching: **Inversion and eversion ankle stretch**

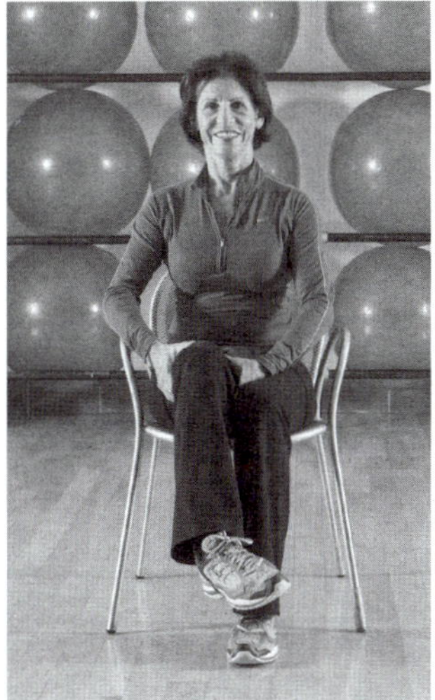

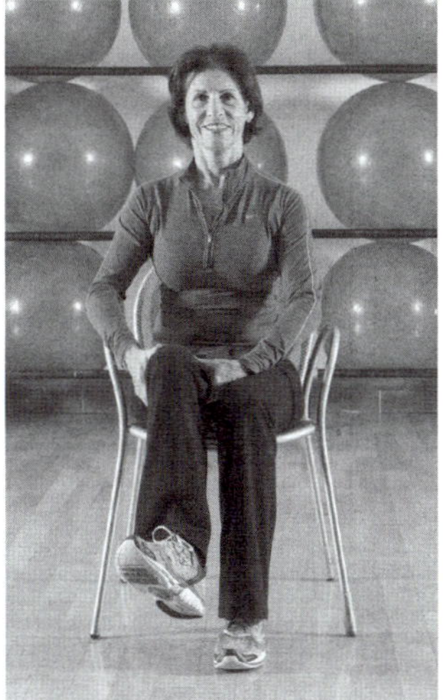

Reps: 3–4 per side
Sets: 1
Intensity: Light
Hold: 10–30 seconds
Rest: No rest needed

Starting position: Sit in a chair with your feet flat on the floor.

Movement: This is a side-to-side movement. Lift your entire right foot a few inches off the floor. Slowly bring the toes of your right foot inward. Hold. Return to center, then slowly bring the toes of your right foot outward. Hold. This is one rep. Finish all reps, then repeat the stretch with your left foot. This completes one set.

Tips and techniques:

- Stretch to the point of mild tension, not pain.
- Maintain neutral posture, with your shoulders down and back.
- Breathe comfortably.

Too hard? Keep your heel grounded on the floor as you turn your foot inward or outward in the stretch.

Too easy? Repeat the stretch several times throughout the day.

12 | Stretching: **Seated point and flex**

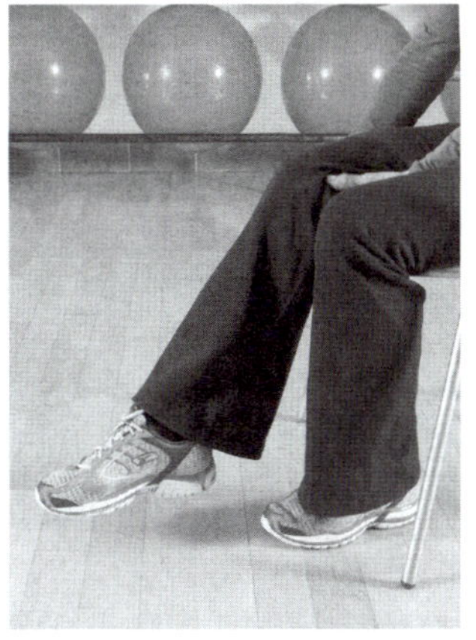

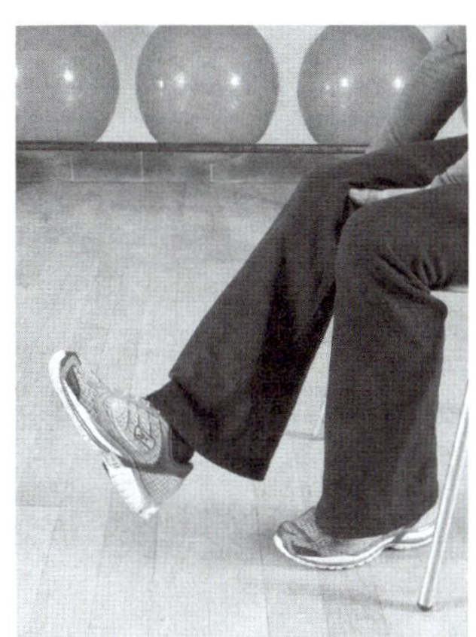

Reps: 3–4 per side
Sets: 1
Intensity: Light
Hold: 10–30 seconds
Rest: No rest needed

Starting position: Sit up straight in a chair with both feet on the floor.

Movement: Lift your right foot a few inches off the floor. Slowly flex your ankle so your toes point up toward the ceiling. Hold. Then slowly point your toes toward the floor. Hold. Finish all reps, then repeat the stretch with your left foot. This completes one set.

Tips and techniques:

- Stretch to the point of mild tension, not pain.
- Maintain neutral posture, with your shoulders down and back.
- Breathe comfortably.

Too hard? Try the stretch while lying on your back with legs extended, so that the backs of your heels touch the floor. Slowly flex your toes and both feet back toward your shin as far as possible. Hold. Slowly point your toes and feet. Hold. This is one rep.

Too easy? Repeat the stretch several times throughout the day.

Note: Special thanks to the Equinox fitness club at 131 Dartmouth Street in Boston for the use of its facilities, and to the following Equinox personal trainers, instructors, and staff members for demonstrating the exercises depicted in this report: Kristy DiScipio, Josie Gardiner, Tracey Knox, and Hector Mancebo.

Knee workout

"Oil me," begged the Tin Woodman haltingly. "Oil me." None of us is made of enough metal to rust in the rain, but creaky, painful knees may make you wish there was such a simple solution. While there isn't a quick fix, there are some things you can do to ease knee pain and build up surrounding muscles so they better support your knee.

Below you'll find brief descriptions of knee anatomy (see Figure 2, below) and joint problems that the knee workout helps ease. The workout itself combines warm-ups, strength exercises to rebuild muscles that help protect your knees, and stretches to release tight tendons, ligaments, and muscles.

Knees 101

The knee is the largest joint in the body. It acts as a hinge that allows your lower leg and foot to swing easily forward or back as you walk, run, or kick. A healthy knee allows almost 150 degrees of movement. But unlike a simple hinge like one on a jewelry box, for example, in which any wobble is undesirable, the knee can slightly rotate or move from side to side, as well. To form the joint, knuckles at the lower end of the thighbone (femur) fit smoothly into dimples in the upper end of the shin bone (tibia) formed by cushioning layers of cartilage called menisci. A quartet of ligaments knits the bones together: a pair of stretchy cruciate ligaments in the interior, and a pair of collateral ligaments on the outer sides of the joint. The kneecap (patella) covers the front of the joint. A large connecting tendon (patellar tendon) bridges the shin, the kneecap, and the large four-part muscle at the front of the thigh called the quadriceps.

Figure 2: Anatomy of the knee

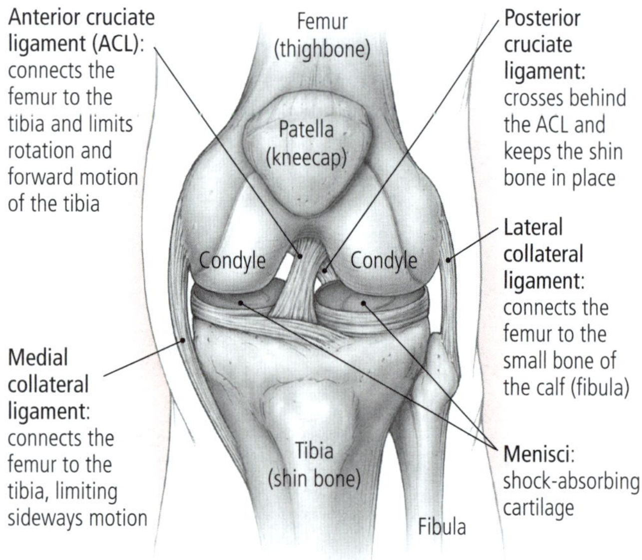

The knee is more than a simple hinge. Along with the strength to raise and lower your body weight, this joint also has supporting structures to allow you to twist and turn.

What this workout helps

Osteoarthritis. This condition is sometimes dubbed "wear and tear" arthritis because it starts when cartilage cushioning the joints wears down (see Figure 3, page 27). Tenderness and morning pain or stiffness that lasts less than 30 minutes are telltale signs of this condition. Osteoarthritis of the knee affects more than four million Americans over the age of 60. Prior injuries, excess weight, aging, and overuse are among the factors that set the stage for knee osteoarthritis. Interestingly, findings from the Framingham Offspring Cohort study suggest that moderately intense exercise like walking or running—at least on normal knees—does not increase the likelihood of osteoarthritis and may even help with treatment.

Bursitis. Small fluid-filled sacs called bursae cushion the movement of bones against muscle, skin, and tendons. Inflammation of a bursa is known as bursitis. Two prime candidates for bursitis lie above and below the knee. Prolonged kneeling while gardening or performing tasks, or sustaining a direct hit to the front of the knee during sports or an accident, can cause bursitis.

Tight hamstring muscles, certain anatomical factors, or actions like repeatedly kicking a ball may play into it, too.

Tendinitis. Marked by pain and swelling above or below the kneecap where tendons attach to bone, tendinitis (inflamed tendons) may have many causes. As you age, protective muscles like the quadriceps weaken and tendons become less flexible. "Weekend warriors" may pay the price for engaging in high-intensity activities like basketball, tennis, or squash without being properly conditioned. Vigorous, repetitive use—or rather overuse—of tendons brought on by dancing, running, or jumping is another possibility.

Runner's knee (patellofemoral pain syndrome). When quadriceps and hamstrings—muscles at the front and back of the thighs—are not sufficiently strong, runners may bend less at the knee while exercising. This funnels pressure to a smaller area, prompting overuse damage that may cause osteoarthritis over time.

Figure 3: Osteoarthritis of the knee

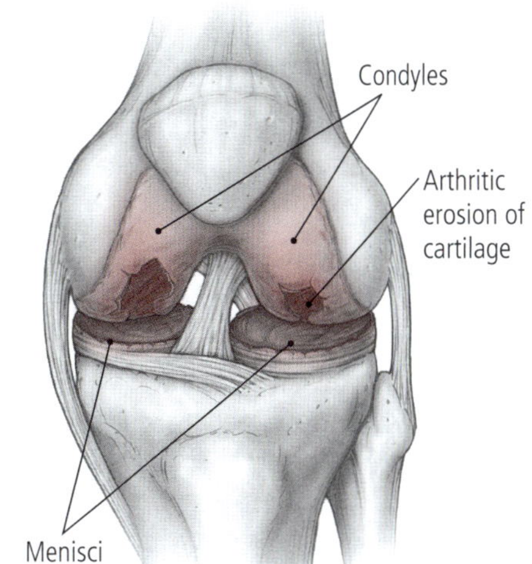

Age, mechanical wear and tear, genetics, and biochemical factors all contribute to the gradual degeneration of the cartilage and the menisci. In this illustration, the cartilage of the condyles (knobs at the lower end of the thighbone) is degraded.

Knee exercises

Strengthening the muscles around the knee and maintaining their power reduces stress across the knee joint. This workout will help you improve flexibility around your knee and build up supporting muscles. If you have osteoarthritis of the knee—a very common complaint as years roll by—doing so will help keep you mobile. Further, building adequate strength and flexibility around the knee makes you less susceptible to bursitis and tendinitis.

We recommend performing the full workout two to three times a week. Make sure you leave 48 hours between strength exercise sessions to allow muscles time to recover. However, warm-ups and stretches can be done daily to further enhance flexibility.

Equipment: Mat, sturdy chair, stability ball, 1- to 3-pound ankle weights (optional), yoga strap (optional).

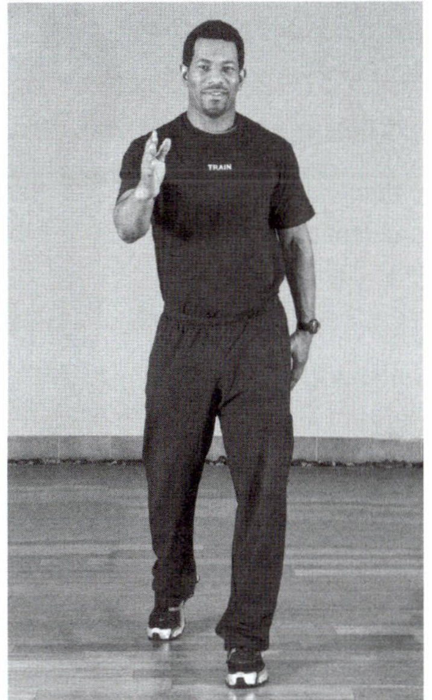

1 | Warming up: Walk forward and back

Reps: 1
Sets: 1–3
Intensity: Light
Tempo: Slow and controlled
Rest: No rest needed

Starting position: Stand up straight with your arms by your sides.

Movement: Walk 10 steps forward. Walk 10 steps backward. This is one rep.

Tips and techniques:

- Maintain neutral posture, with your shoulders down and back.
- Let your arms swing naturally forward and back.

2 | Warming up: **Mini-squats**

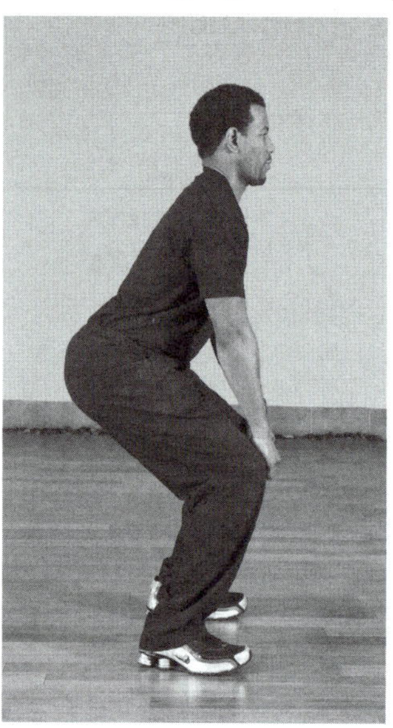

Reps: 10
Sets: 1–3
Intensity: Moderate
Tempo: Slow and controlled
Rest: No rest needed

Starting position: Stand up straight with your feet hip-width apart.

Movement: Rest your hands on your thighs. Hinge forward at your hips and bend your knees to lower your buttocks about six inches, as if starting to sit down in a chair. Keep your heels down and make sure your knees do not extend in front of your toes. Return to the starting position. This is one rep.

Tips and techniques:

- Press your weight back into your heels when squatting.
- Keep your knees aligned over your feet and pointing forward as you squat.
- Keep your spine neutral and your shoulders down and back.

Too hard? Do a smaller squat.
Too easy? Hold each mini-squat for eight counts.

3 | Warming up: **Alternating hamstring curls**

Reps: 10
Sets: 1–3
Intensity: Light
Tempo: Slow and controlled
Rest: No rest needed

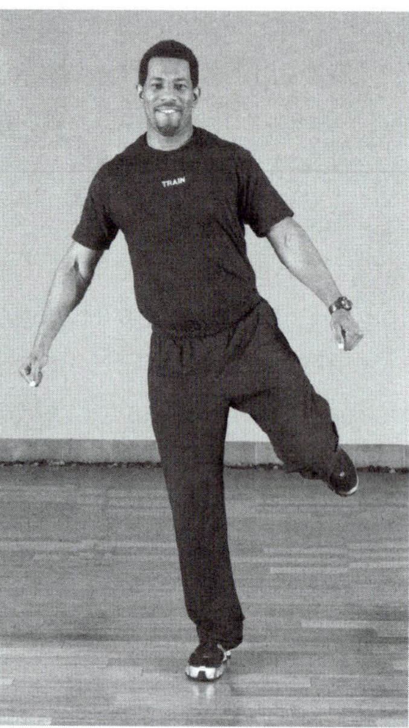

Starting position: Stand up straight with your feet hip-width apart.

Movement: Lift your right heel toward your buttocks and return to the starting position, then lift your left heel toward your buttocks and return to the starting position. This is one rep.

Tips and techniques:

- Maintain neutral posture, with your shoulders down and back.
- Contract your abdominal muscles.
- Breathe naturally.

Too hard? Do not lift your heels as high.
Too easy? Add a little squat between lifts.

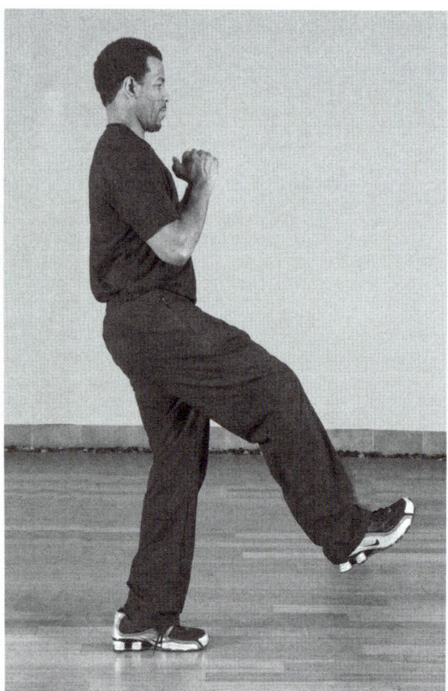

4 | Warming up: **Standing single leg circles**

Reps: 10 per leg
Sets: 1–3
Intensity: Light
Tempo: Slow and controlled
Rest: No rest needed

Starting position: Stand up straight with your feet hip-width apart.

Movement: Lift your right foot off the floor and move it in a circle as if pedaling a bike. Finish all reps, then return to the starting position. Repeat with the left foot. This completes one set.

Tips and techniques:

- Maintain neutral posture, with your shoulders down and back.
- Be sure to contract the buttock muscles in the standing hip for stability.
- Contract your abdominal muscles to avoid leaning backward.

Too hard? Hold on to a chair or counter for support.
Too easy? Try not to touch the floor as you make each circular motion.

5 | Strengthening: **Supine knee extension**

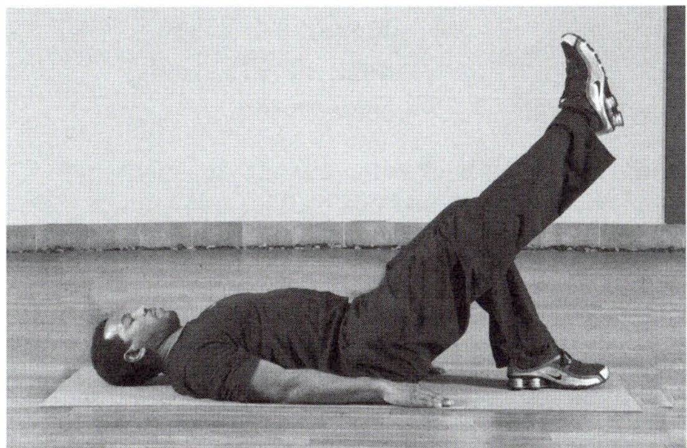

Reps: 10 per leg
Sets: 1–3
Intensity: Light to moderate
Tempo: 3-1-3
Rest: 30–90 seconds between sets

Starting position: Lie on a mat on your back with both knees bent and feet flat on the floor. Rest your arms at your sides.

Movement: Slowly lift your right foot off the floor and straighten your leg while keeping your knees level. Pause, then slowly lower your foot to the starting position so that both feet are flat on the floor. Finish all reps, then repeat with the left foot. This completes one set.

Tips and techniques:

- As you lift your foot, straighten your leg as much as possible without locking the knee.
- Maintain a neutral posture, with your shoulders down and back.
- Exhale as you lift.

Too hard? Lift your foot a shorter distance.
Too easy? Add a 1- to 3-pound ankle weight.

6 | Strengthening: **Seated knee extension**

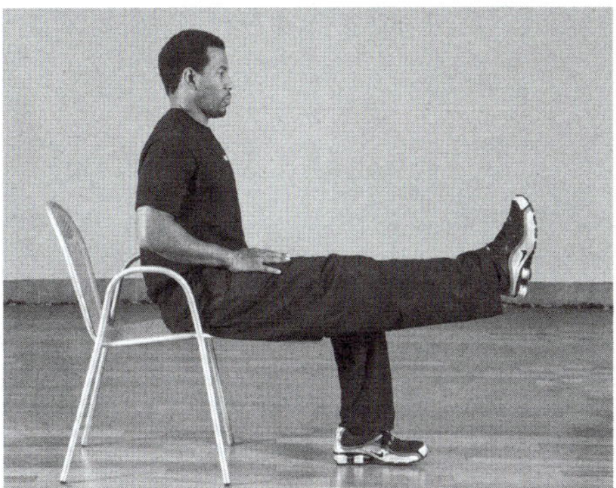

Reps: 10 per leg
Sets: 1–3
Intensity: Light to moderate
Tempo: 3-1-3
Rest: 30–90 seconds between sets

Starting position: Sit up straight on a chair or bench with your feet flat on the floor and your hands resting on your thighs.

Movement: Slowly lift up your right foot to the level of your hip. Pause, then slowly lower the foot to the starting position (flat on the floor). Finish all reps, then repeat with the left leg. This completes one set.

Tips and techniques:

- Maintain neutral posture, with your shoulders down and back.
- Lift your leg as high as possible without locking your knee.
- Exhale as you lift.

Too hard? Lift your foot a shorter distance.
Too easy? Add a 1- to 3-pound ankle weight.

7 | Strengthening: **Chair stand with staggered legs**

Reps: 10 per leg
Sets: 1–3
Intensity: Moderate to hard
Tempo: 3-1-3
Rest: 30–90 seconds between sets

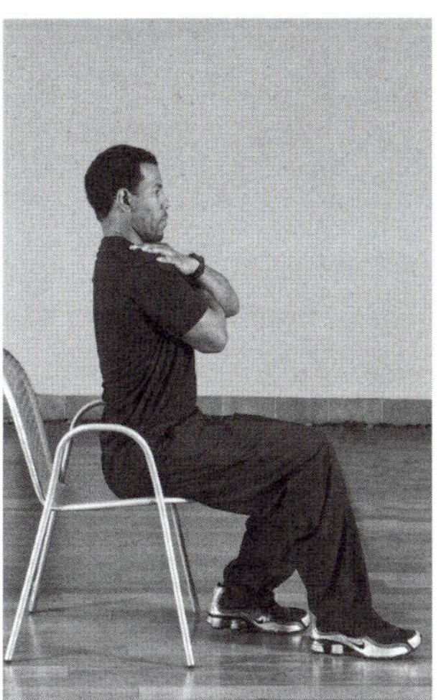

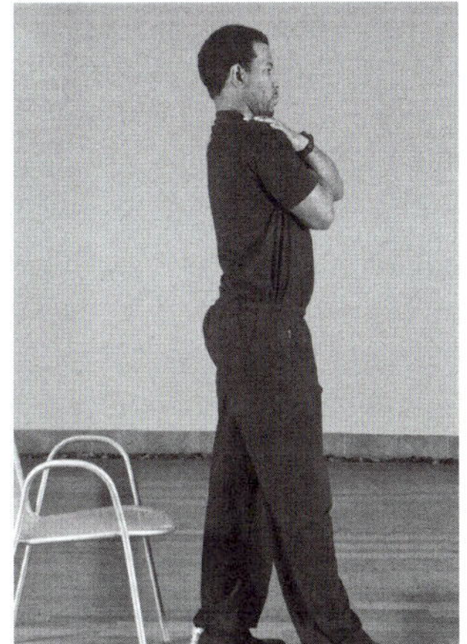

Starting position: Sit up straight near the front edge of a chair with your arms crossed and fingers touching opposite shoulders. Position your feet hip-width apart and stagger them by moving your right foot forward.

Movement: Smoothly stand up with your knees and hips pointing straight ahead. Pause, then return to the starting position. Finish all reps, then repeat with the left foot forward. This completes one set.

Tips and techniques:

- Maintain neutral posture throughout the movement.
- Tighten the muscles in your abdomen and buttocks.
- Exhale as you lift up.

Too hard? Line up your feet evenly, hip-width apart, in the starting position.
Too easy? Lift your arms over your head. Keep your shoulders down and back throughout the move.

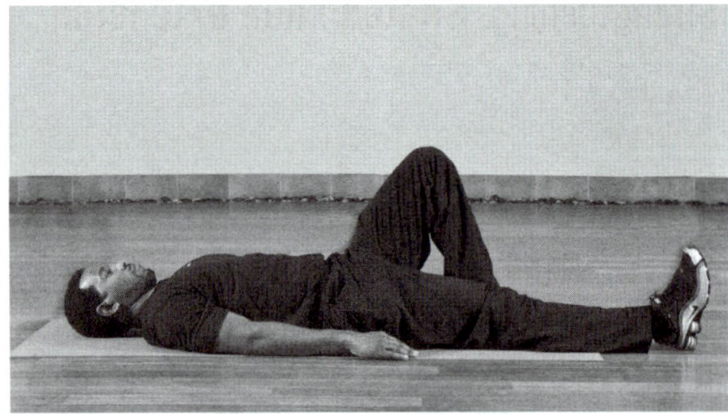

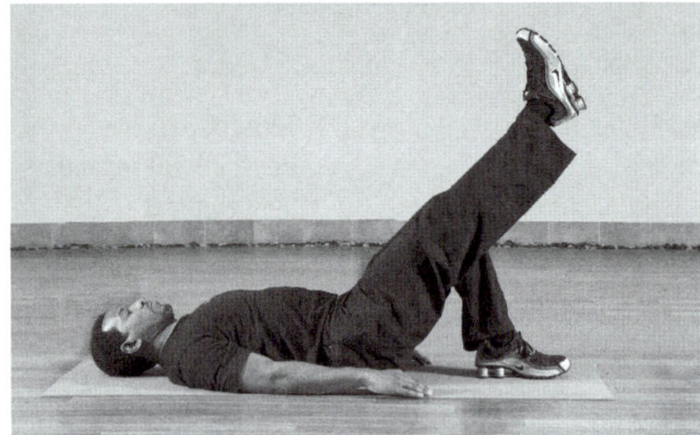

8 | Strengthening: **Single leg lift**

Reps: 10 per leg
Sets: 1–3
Intensity: Light to moderate
Tempo: 3-1-3
Rest: 30–90 seconds between sets

Starting position: Lie on your back with your left knee bent and foot flat on the floor. Extend your right leg. Rest your hands by your hips on the floor.

Movement: Tighten your thigh muscles and slowly lift your right leg in the air until the knees are aligned. Pause, then slowly lower your leg to rest on the floor. Finish all reps, then repeat with the left leg. This completes one set.

Tips and techniques:

- Maintain a neutral posture, with your shoulders down and back.
- Be sure to tighten your thigh muscle before lifting the leg.
- Exhale as you lift.

Too hard? Lift your leg a shorter distance.

Too easy? Try doing the leg lift in the shape of a T at a slow, controlled pace. Lift up your right leg 4 inches, move the leg toward your left leg 4 inches, return to center, move the leg 4 inches to the right, return to center, then lower your leg to the floor. Finish all reps, repeat with the left leg. This completes one set.

9 | Strengthening: **Wall squats with stability ball**

Reps: 10
Sets: 1–3
Intensity: Moderate to hard
Tempo: 3-1-3
Rest: 30–90 seconds between sets

Starting position: Stand up straight and place the stability ball between the back of your waist and the wall. Walk your feet out about 18 to 24 inches, while keeping the ball at waist height. Rest your hands on your thighs.

Movement: Slowly bend your knees and hips into a squat as if you were sitting down in a chair. (The ball will roll up your back as you move downward.) Stop before your buttocks reach knee level. Slowly straighten your legs as you return to the starting position. This is one rep.

Tips and techniques:

- Maintain neutral posture, with your shoulders down and back.
- Keep your knees aligned over your ankles and pointing forward as you squat.
- Exhale as you return to the starting position.

Too hard? Do a smaller squat.

Too easy? Hold each squat for eight counts.

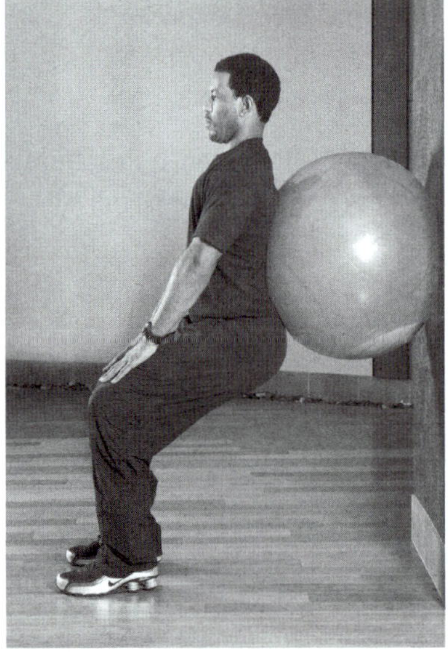

10 | Stretching: **Quadriceps stretch on stomach**

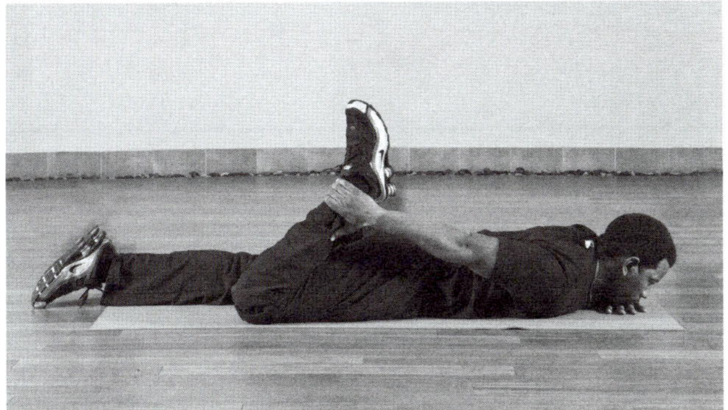

Reps: 3–4 per leg
Sets: 1
Intensity: Moderate
Hold: 10–30 seconds
Rest: No rest needed

Starting position: Lie on your stomach on the floor with your hands flat under your chin.

Movement: Bend your right knee and try to bring the heel toward your right buttock. Reach back with your right hand and take hold of your foot. Hold the stretch, then slowly lower your foot to the floor. Repeat the stretch with your left leg. Continue alternating legs until you finish all reps.

Tips and techniques:

- Stretch to the point of mild tension, not pain.
- Breathe comfortably.

Too hard? Place a yoga strap around your foot to assist with the stretch.

Too easy? Lift your knee up slightly off the floor to increase the stretch.

11 | Stretching: **Alternating hamstring stretch**

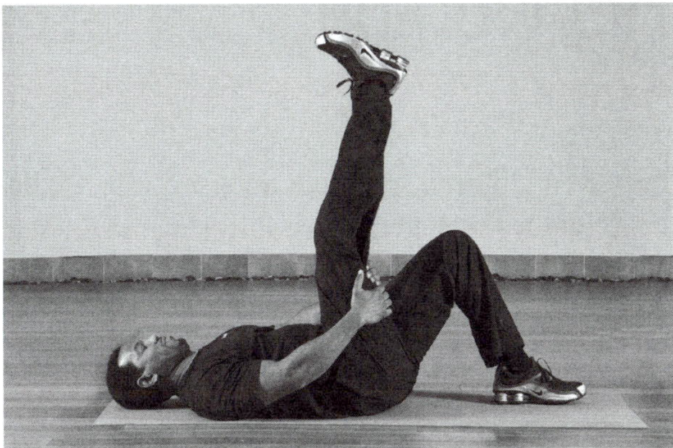

Reps: 3–4
Sets: 1
Intensity: Moderate to hard
Hold: 10–30 seconds
Rest: No rest needed

Starting position:
Lie on your back with both knees bent and feet flat on the floor.

Movement: Grasp your right leg with both hands behind the thigh. Extend your leg to lift your right foot toward the ceiling. Straighten the leg as much as possible without locking the knee and flex the ankle to stretch the calf muscles. Hold. Return to the starting position and repeat with the left leg. This is one rep.

Tips and techniques:

- Stretch the leg extended toward the ceiling to the point of mild tension without any pressure behind the knee or any pain.
- Relax your shoulders down and back into the floor.
- Breathe comfortably.

Too hard? Sit up straight in a chair and extend your right leg straight out in front of you with the heel grounded on the floor and the toes pointing to the ceiling. Hinge forward from the hip while maintaining a neutral spine. Hold. Repeat with the left leg. This is one rep.

Too easy? Stand upright and extend your right leg straight in front of you with your foot on a chair or counter. Flex your ankle. Hinge forward from the hip while maintaining a neutral spine. Hold. Repeat with the left leg. This is one rep.

Hip workout

Ever seen children spin hula hoops in easy, endless circles? Or watched the tiny, shivering moves made by a belly dancer with one hip aslant? Remember doing the Twist? Then you know that hips are capable of far more than most of us manage in the course of our daily rounds. If you have hip pain, you may not be salsa dancing anytime soon, but by conditioning the muscles that help support your hip, you may find that you can perform physical activities and everyday tasks more easily and painlessly.

This section includes brief descriptions of hip anatomy (see Figure 4, at right) and joint and muscle problems that the hip workout helps ease. The workout moves from warm-ups to strength exercises aimed at rebuilding muscles that help protect your hips. Stretches help release tight tendons and muscles that affect gait and balance and may play a role in back pain, too.

Figure 4: Anatomy of the hip

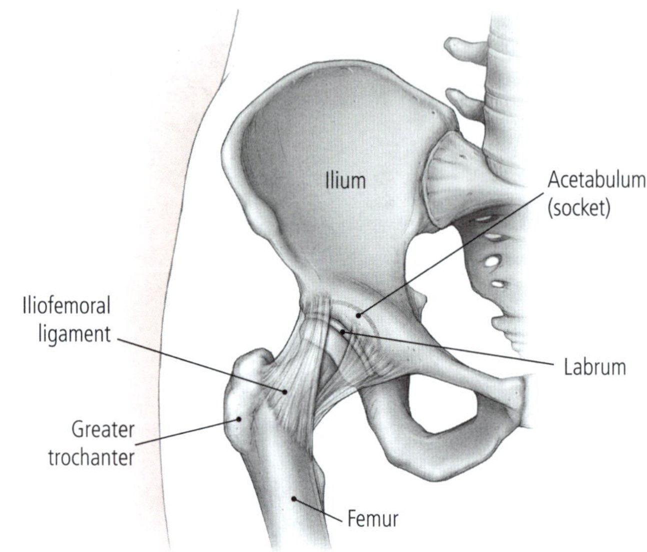

The hip is a ball-and-socket joint reinforced by a strong ring of cartilage (labrum) inside the socket (acetabulum). Supporting ligaments allow for a wide range of motion while the hip bears the full weight of the upper body.

Hips 101

The hip joint is a ball-and-socket design, albeit one with far less flexibility than the shoulder joint. Three fused bones—the ischium, ilium, and pubis—shape the basin of the pelvis. At the neck of the thighbone (femur), a bump branches off to form the ball of the hip joint with its cushioning layer of cartilage. The ball fits snugly into a socket in the pelvis (acetabulum). Thanks to the perfect fit, along with the slick cartilage coating the bones and the fluid lubricating the space between them, the friction between the ball and socket in a healthy hip is less than that of two ice cubes rubbing together. A larger projection slightly lower on the thighbone provides an anchor for tendons that run into leg and hip muscles, while a series of ligaments tightly bind the joint to help provide stability.

What this workout helps

Osteoarthritis. Sometimes dubbed "wear and tear" arthritis because it starts when cartilage cushioning the joints wears down, osteoarthritis of the hip affects one in four American adults during their lives. The joint space narrows and the cartilage thins as bones rub against it, or eventually against each other, sometimes to the point of creating rough spots or bone spurs. Marked by pain in the groin or down the leg, this condition may go unreported because people sometimes assume that the knee, rather than the hip, is the problem. Prior injuries, excess weight, aging, and overuse are among the factors that set the stage for hip osteoarthritis.

Poor balance. Muscles known as hip flexors allow you to bend at the hip and bring your knee up toward your chest. Often, these muscles grow tight and shorten, tugging your upper body forward. This affects balance and gait while walking.

Back pain. Short, tight hip flexors contribute to lower back pain, particularly when the iliopsoas muscles, which balance your pelvis, are tight, too.

Hip exercises

By enhancing hip flexibility and strengthening supporting muscles, this workout improves balance and makes walking easier. It also helps address pain and reduced mobility from osteoarthritis of the hip, as well as back pain.

We recommend performing the full workout two to three times a week. Make sure you leave 48 hours between strength exercise sessions to allow muscles time to recover. However, warm-ups and stretches can be done daily, if you wish, to further enhance flexibility.

Equipment: Mat, stability ball, yoga strap, sturdy chair (optional), resistance tubing (optional), 1- to 3-pound ankle weights (optional).

1 | Warming up: **Alternating knee lifts**

Reps: 10
Sets: 1
Intensity: Light
Tempo: Slow and controlled
Rest: No rest needed

Starting position: Stand up straight with your feet together and your hands at your sides.

Movement: Shift weight onto your left leg and lift your right knee toward the ceiling. Lower to the starting position. Repeat with your left knee. This is one rep.

Tips and techniques:

- Keep your chest lifted and your shoulders down and back.
- Contract your abdominal muscles throughout to avoid leaning backward.

Too hard? Hold on to a chair for support.
Too easy? Do 10 knee lifts on the right side, then 10 on the left, to complete one set.

2 | Warming up: **Hip circles on back**

Reps: 20 per leg (10 in each direction)
Sets: 1
Intensity: Light
Tempo: Slow and controlled
Rest: No rest needed

Starting position: Lie on your back with your left knee bent and the foot flat on the floor. Place a yoga strap over the foot of the right leg and extend it.

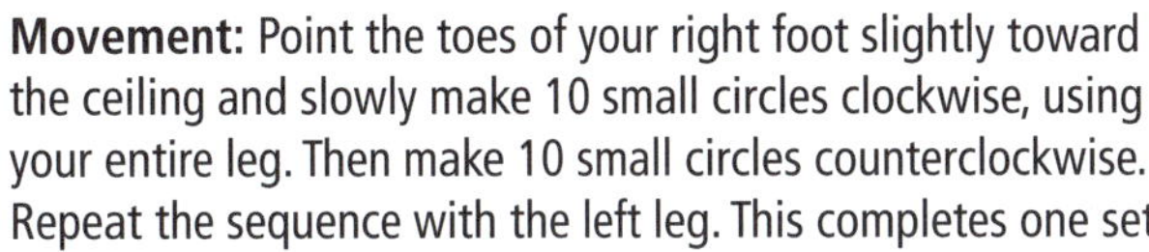

Movement: Point the toes of your right foot slightly toward the ceiling and slowly make 10 small circles clockwise, using your entire leg. Then make 10 small circles counterclockwise. Repeat the sequence with the left leg. This completes one set.

Tips and techniques:

- Initiate the movement from the hip.
- Contract your abdominal muscles and be sure your back is touching the floor throughout.

Too hard? Make smaller circles to limit your range of motion.
Too easy? Make larger circles.

3 | Warming up: **Hip circles on stability ball**

Reps: 10 in each direction
Sets: 1
Intensity: Light
Tempo: Slow and controlled
Rest: No rest needed

Starting position: Sit on a stability ball with your feet hip-width apart. Place your hands next to your hips on the ball for extra support.

Movement: Move your hips in a slow clockwise circle to loosen up your hip joints, keeping your buttocks on the ball as you do so. Finish all reps, then repeat the circles counterclockwise. This completes one set.

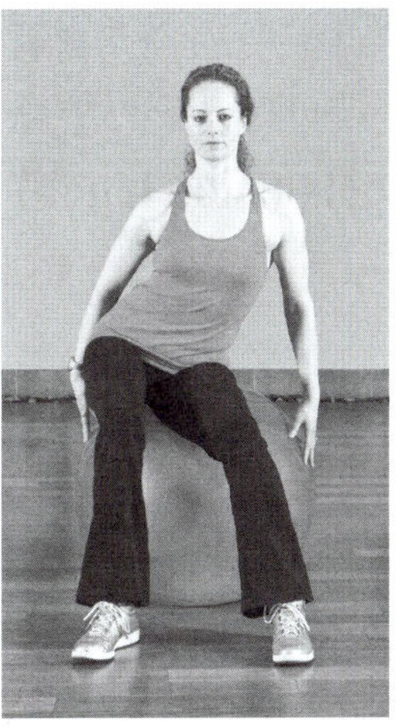

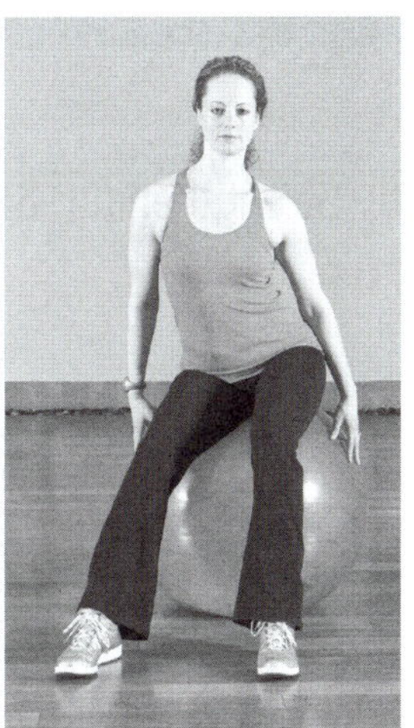

Tips and techniques:

- Keep your shoulders down and back.
- Contract your abdominal muscles throughout.
- Keep your pace slow and controlled.

Too hard? Perform hip circles standing upright with knees slightly bent.
Too easy? Perform the exercise without holding on to the ball.

4 | Strengthening: **Side-lying clam**

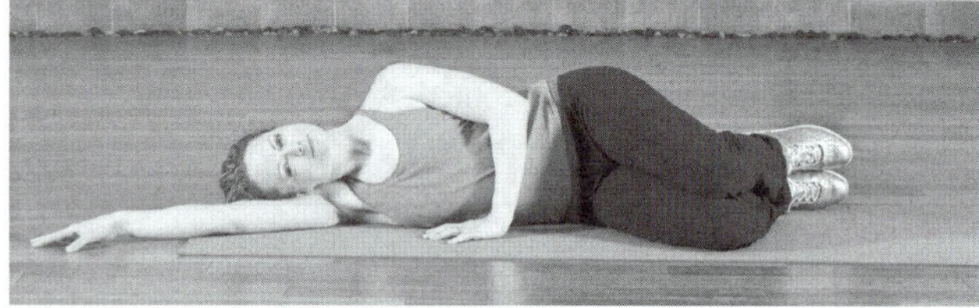

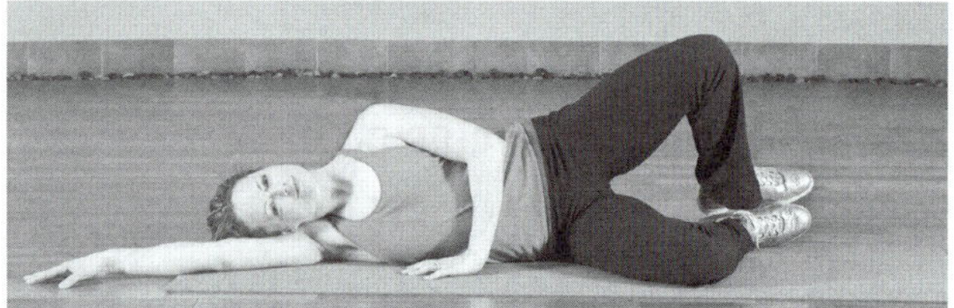

Reps: 10 per side
Sets: 1–3
Intensity: Light to moderate
Tempo: 3-1-3
Rest: 30–90 seconds between sets

Starting position: Lie on your right side, knees bent so your heels are in line with your buttocks. Rest your head on your right arm on the floor.

Movement: Keep your feet together as you slowly lift your left knee up toward the ceiling. Pause, then slowly return to the starting position. Finish all reps, then repeat on the left side. This completes one set.

Tips and techniques:

- Throughout the movement, keep your hips stacked and still as if you were lying with your back against a wall.
- Lift your top knee up as high as possible without letting your hip move.
- Exhale as you lift.

Too hard? Lift your top knee a shorter distance or lean your back against a wall for support.

Too easy? Tie resistance tubing around your upper thighs, or increase the number of reps.

5 | Strengthening: **Wall squats with stability ball**

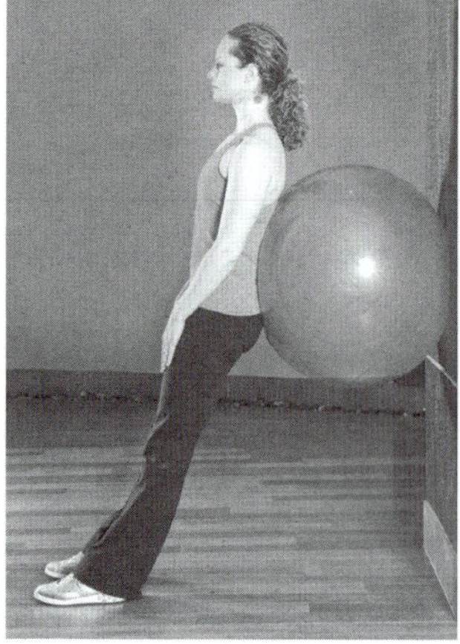

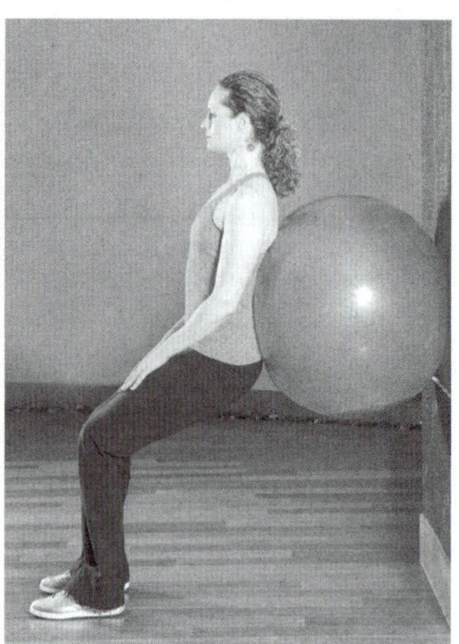

Reps: 10
Sets: 1–3
Intensity: Moderate
Tempo: 3-1-3
Rest: 30–90 seconds between sets

Starting position: Stand up straight and place the stability ball between the back of your waist and the wall. Walk your feet out about 18 to 24 inches, while keeping the ball at waist height. Rest your hands on your thighs.

Movement: Slowly bend your knees and hips into a squat as if you were sitting down in a chair. (The ball will roll up your back as you move downward.) Stop before your buttocks reach knee level. Straighten your legs as you return to the starting position. This is one rep.

Tips and techniques:

- Maintain neutral posture, with your shoulders down and back.
- Keep your knees aligned over your ankles and pointing forward as you squat.
- Exhale as you return to the starting position.

Too hard? Do a smaller squat.

Too easy? Hold each squat for eight counts.

6 | Strengthening: **Standing side leg lift**

Reps: 10 per leg
Sets: 1–3
Intensity: Moderate
Tempo: 3-1-3
Rest: 30–90 seconds between sets

Starting position: Stand up straight with your feet together and your hands on your hips.

Movement: Slowly lift your left leg straight out to the side. Pause, then slowly lower the leg. Keep your hips even throughout. Finish all reps, then repeat with the right leg. This completes one set.

Tips and techniques:

- Maintain neutral posture, with your shoulders down and back.
- Tighten your abdominal muscles and squeeze the buttocks of your supporting leg.
- Exhale as you lift.

Too hard? Hold on to the back of a chair for balance and lift your leg a shorter distance.

Too easy? Hold for four counts at the top of the lift during each rep.

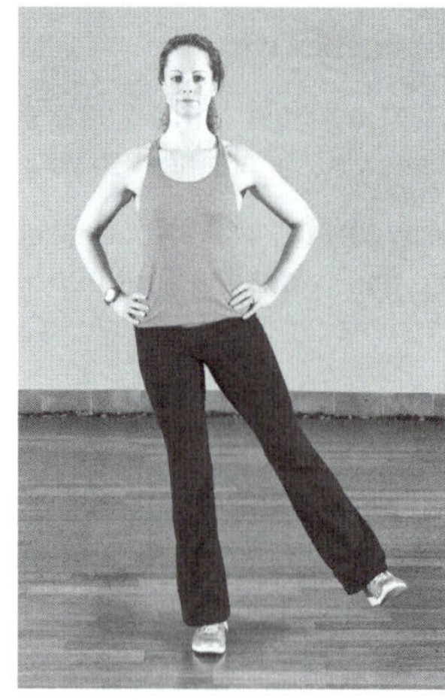

7 | Strengthening: **Bridge with alternating single leg lift**

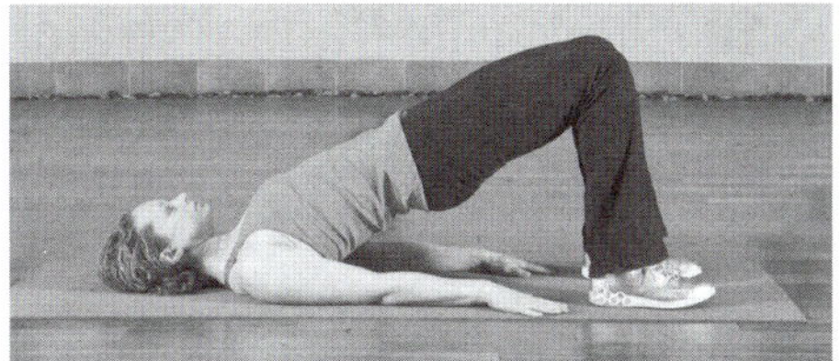

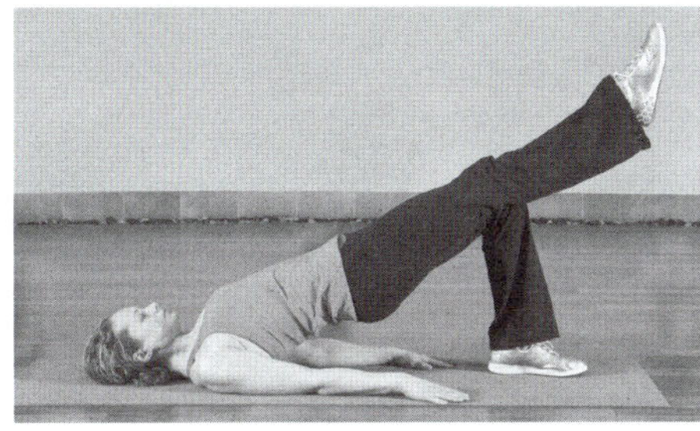

Reps: 5 per leg
Sets: 1–3
Intensity: Moderate
Tempo: 2-2-2-2
Rest: 30–90 seconds between sets

Starting position: Lie on your back on the floor with your knees bent and feet flat on the floor, hip-width apart. Place your arms at your sides. Relax your shoulders down and back against the floor.

Movement: Squeeze your buttocks as you lift your hips off the floor to a count of two. This is the bridge position. Lift the right foot and extend your leg out to the height of the bent knee to a count of two. Bring the right foot back to the floor into the bridge position to a count of two, then return to the starting position (hips on the floor) to a count of two. Repeat with the left leg. Continue alternating legs until you finish all reps. This completes one set.

Tips and techniques:

- Be sure to squeeze your buttocks before you lift up into bridge position.
- Keep your shoulders, hips, and knees aligned.
- Relax your shoulders down and back into the floor.

Too hard? Perform the bridge without the leg extension, using a 2-1-2 count (lifting your hips up to a count of two, holding for one second, and returning your hips to the floor to a count of two).
Too easy? Cross your arms on your chest.

8 | Strengthening: **Quadruped single leg lift**

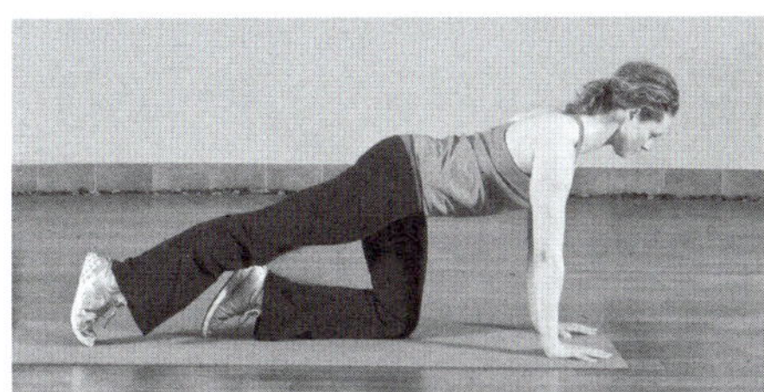

Reps: 10 per side
Sets: 1–3
Intensity: Light to moderate
Tempo: 3-1-3
Rest: 30–90 seconds between sets

Starting position: Position yourself on hands and knees ("all fours") on the floor.

Movement: Extend your right leg behind you, slowly lifting it up to hip level. Pause, then return to the starting position. Finish all reps, then repeat with your left leg. This completes one set.

Tips and techniques:

- Keep your shoulders and hips even.
- Maintain a neutral spine.
- Contract your abdominal muscles throughout to avoid letting your stomach drop and your back arch.

Too hard? Lie on your stomach, resting your chin on your hands. Slowly lift one leg off the floor. Pause, then return to the starting position. Finish all reps, then repeat with the opposite leg.
Too easy? Add 1- to 3-pound ankle weights.

9 | Stretching: **Kneeling hip flexor stretch**

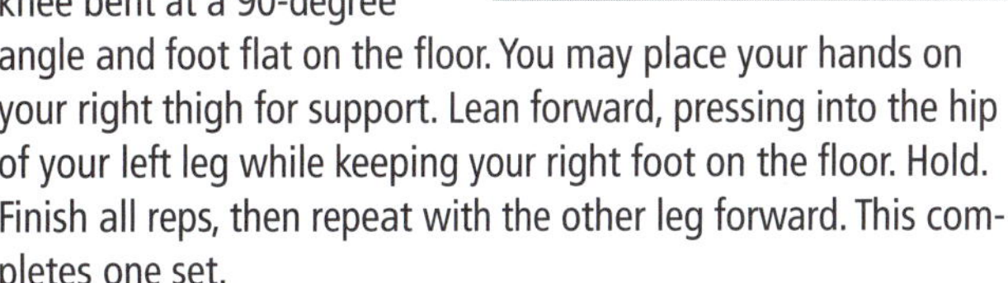

Reps: 3–4 per side
Sets: 1
Intensity: Moderate
Hold: 10–30 seconds
Rest: No rest needed

Starting position: Kneel on the mat.

Movement: Put your right leg in front of you with the knee bent at a 90-degree angle and foot flat on the floor. You may place your hands on your right thigh for support. Lean forward, pressing into the hip of your left leg while keeping your right foot on the floor. Hold. Finish all reps, then repeat with the other leg forward. This completes one set.

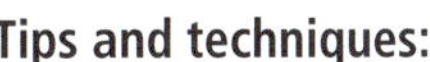

Tips and techniques:

- Stretch to the point of mild tension, not pain. Feel the stretch in the crease of the back leg.
- Maintain a neutral spine while keeping hips and shoulders even.
- Keep your shoulders down and back, and your abdominal muscles contracted.

Too hard? Lie on your back. Pull your right knee toward your chest and extend your left leg on the floor. Flex your left foot and press your left calf down into the floor. You'll feel this stretch at the front of the extended leg, the lower back, and the buttock of the bent knee. Hold. Finish all reps, then switch legs to repeat.
Too easy? As you lean forward, pressing into the hip of your left leg, lift your left arm up and over as if raising your hand in class.

10 | Stretching: **Gluteal stretch**

Reps: 3–4
Sets: 1
Intensity: Moderate
Hold: 10–30 seconds
Rest: No rest needed

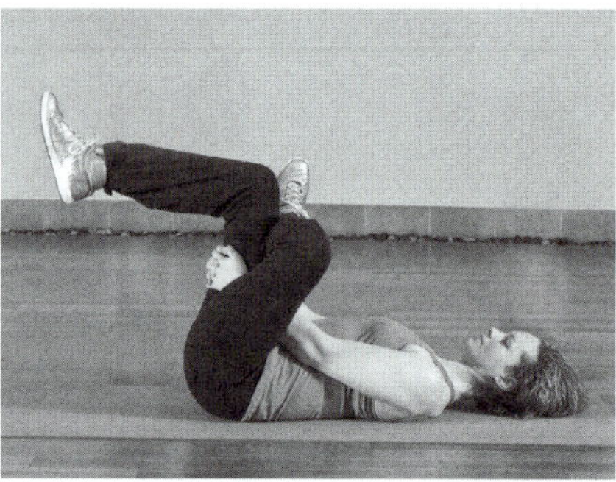

Starting position: Lie on your back with your right knee bent and your foot on the floor. Rest your left ankle on your right kneecap. Your left knee should point toward the wall.

Movement: Hold the back of the right thigh with both hands and slowly lift your right foot up off the floor until you feel the stretch in your left hip and buttock. Hold. Return to the starting position, then repeat on the opposite side. This is one rep. Continue alternating leg positions until you finish all reps.

Tips and techniques:

- Stretch to the point of mild tension, not pain.
- Relax your shoulders down and back into the floor.
- Breathe comfortably.

Too hard? Lie on your back with both knees bent and your feet flat on the floor. Cross your right knee over your left knee and pull your knees in toward your chest. Repeat with your left knee crossed over your right knee. This is one rep.

Too easy? Lie on your back with your right knee bent and your foot on the floor. Rest your left ankle on your right kneecap. Clasp your right knee with both hands and lift your right foot up off the floor. Repeat with your right ankle on your left kneecap. This is one rep.

11 | Stretching: **Butterfly pose**

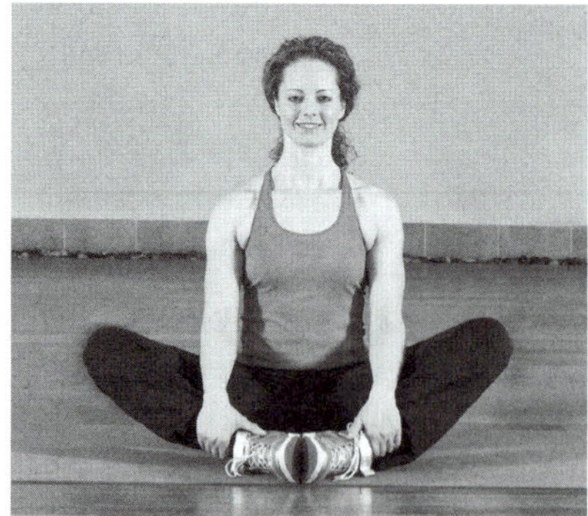

Reps: 3–4
Sets: 1
Intensity: Moderate
Hold: 10–30 seconds
Rest: No rest needed

Starting position: Sit on the floor. Bring the soles of your feet together and let your knees fall apart toward the floor.

Movement: Place your hands on your ankles. Hinge forward from your hips until you feel the stretch in your inner thighs. Hold. Return to the starting position. This is one rep.

Tips and techniques:

- Stretch to the point of mild tension, not pain.
- Maintain a neutral head and spine with your shoulders down and back and abdominal muscles contracted.
- Breathe comfortably.

Too hard? Perform the stretch while lying on your back, pulling your feet toward you with knees out to the side.

Too easy? Sit against a wall and pull in your feet for a greater stretch.

12 | Stretching: **Hamstring stretch**

Reps: 3–4
Sets: 1
Intensity: Moderate
Hold: 10–30 seconds
Rest: No rest needed

Starting position: Lie on your back with both knees bent and feet flat on the floor.

Movement: Hold your right leg with both hands behind the thigh. Lift your right foot toward the ceiling as you extend your knee. Straighten the leg as much as possible without locking the knee. As you do so, flex the ankle to stretch the calf muscles. Hold. Repeat with the left leg. This is one rep. Continue alternating leg positions until you finish all reps.

Tips and techniques:

- Stretch the leg extended toward the ceiling to the point of mild tension without any pressure behind the knee or any pain.
- Relax your shoulders down and back into the floor.
- Breathe comfortably.

Too hard? Sit up straight in a chair and extend one leg straight out in front of you with the toes pointing to the ceiling. Hinge forward from the hip while maintaining a neutral spine. Finish all reps, then repeat with other leg.

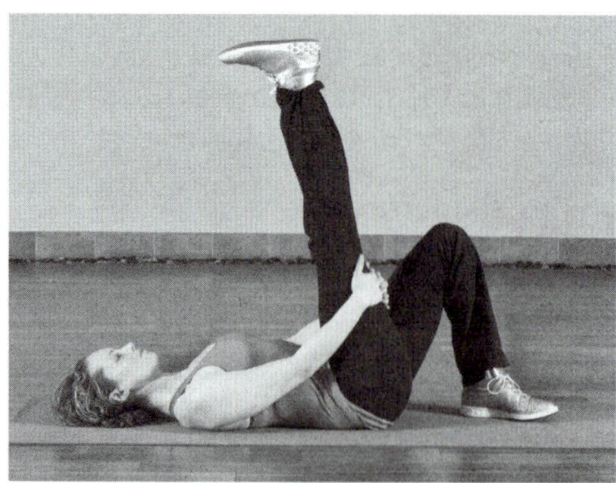

Too easy? Stand upright and extend one leg straight in front of you with your foot on a chair or counter. Flex your ankle. Hinge forward from the hip while maintaining a neutral spine. Finish all reps, then repeat with other leg.

Shoulder workout

While busy hands often get all the credit, the most mundane daily tasks—brushing your hair, sweeping your wallet off the dresser, reaching for the front doorknob—can't be done unless your shoulders position your arms and hands in the right spots.

Shoulders 101

Although we refer to the shoulder as if it were a single joint, in reality four joints loosely connect several bones. Riding above the rib cage are four bones that form the shoulder girdle: a pair of collarbones (clavicles) at the front, and a pair of triangular shoulder blades or wing bones (scapulae) at the back. The inner end of each collarbone is linked to the breastbone (sternum). The outer end of the collarbone fits into a small joint meeting up with the front edge of the shoulder blade (forming the acromioclavicular, or AC, joint), so that the four bones largely float above the ribs, suspended by several strong muscles and ligaments.

The long bone of the upper arm (humerus) fits into a larger ball-and-socket joint at the shoulder blade (see Figure 5, at right). This allows the arm to move freely in many directions, making it possible to serve a tennis ball or push a vacuum. Yet it also makes the shoulder joint inherently unstable and easy to injure.

A tendon bridging four small muscles creates the rotator cuff. The cuff covers the ball of the shoulder joint and permits you to rotate your arm and stabilizes the joint. Even a basic action, like lifting your arm, requires every part of the shoulder girdle to move in turn and calls into play rotator cuff muscles plus a raft of strong muscles of the shoulders, back, and chest.

What this workout helps

Shoulder impingement. A common cause of shoulder pain occurs when the front portion of the shoulder blade impinges on the rotator cuff as you raise your arm. This may cause bursitis or tendinitis or a tear in the rotator cuff. Shoulder impingement causes pain and limits movement considerably, occasionally creating a "frozen shoulder." Common causes include overuse of rotator cuff muscles in sports like tennis, swimming, and baseball, work like painting that repeatedly involves reaching overhead, and minor injuries.

Osteoarthritis. Sometimes dubbed "wear and tear" arthritis because it starts when cartilage cushioning the joints wears down, osteoarthritis of the shoulder is a common cause of pain in people over age 50. Prior injuries, aging, and overuse are all factors.

Bursitis. Small, fluid-filled sacs called bursae cushion the movement of bones against muscle, skin, and tendons. Bursae above the rotator cuff are prime candidates for inflammation (bursitis) prompted by causes similar to those for shoulder impingement or because of anatomical factors.

Tendinitis. Shoulder impingement may lead to pain, swelling, and inflammation of the rotator cuff tendon.

Figure 5: Anatomy of the shoulder joint

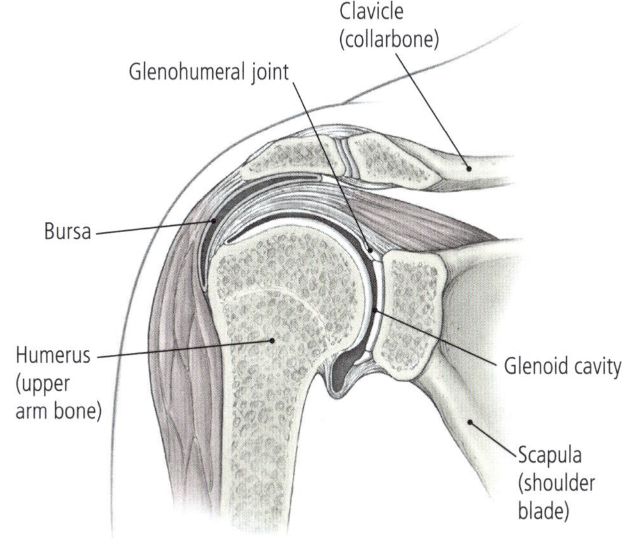

Many shoulder injuries involve the shoulder's main joint, where the humerus connects with the shoulder socket (called the glenoid) at the scapula.

Shoulder exercises

As the least stable joint in your body, your shoulders will benefit from exercises designed to strengthen supporting muscles while gently increasing your range of motion, so that you can easily swing a golf club or reach overhead, for example. Impingements that prevent movements like these are often a result of poor shoulder flexibility and impaired movement patterns. Maintaining strength and flexibility in your shoulder also reduces stress across the joint, making you less susceptible to bursitis and tendinitis.

For the first two weeks: Do only the warm-ups and stretches. Practice at least two to three times a week or as often as daily.

Starting at week 3: Begin to perform the full workout two to three times a week. Make sure you leave 48 hours between strength exercise sessions to allow muscles time to recover. Warm-ups and stretches can be done daily to further enhance flexibility.

Equipment: 1- to 3-pound hand weights, resistance tubing with door attachment, stability ball, hand towel.

1 | Warming up: **Shoulder circles**

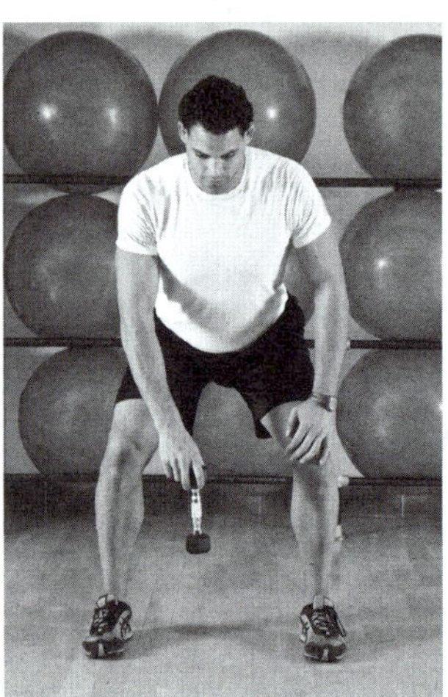

Reps: 20 per arm (10 in each direction)
Sets: 1
Intensity: Light
Tempo: Slow and controlled
Rest: No rest needed

Starting position: Stand up straight with your feet hip-width apart. Hold a 1- to 3-pound weight in your right hand with one end of the weight hanging down toward the floor.

Movement: Bend your knees a bit and slightly hinge forward from the hip so that you're holding the weight between your legs. You can rest your left hand on your left thigh for support. Make 10 clockwise circles with your right arm as if stirring a pot. Pause, then reverse direction for 10 circles. Move the weight to your left hand and repeat the sequence. This completes one set.

Tips and techniques:

- Hinge from the hips without bending or arching your back.
- Maintain a neutral spine, and keep your shoulders down and back.
- Allow the weight to hang like a dead weight.

Too hard? Perform the exercise while seated, or try it standing with no weight.

Too easy? Make a larger circle.

2 | Warming up: **Shoulder pendulums**

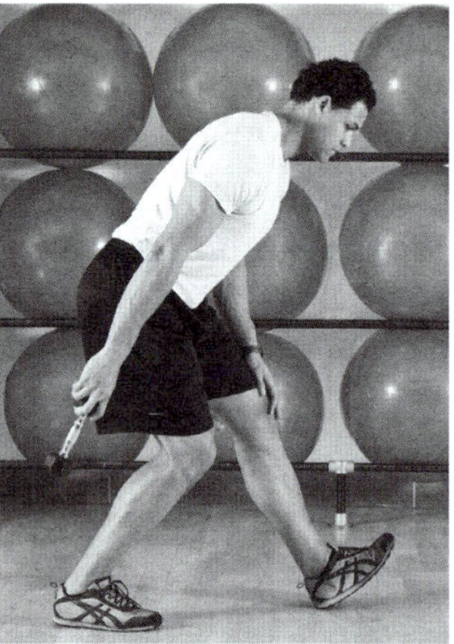

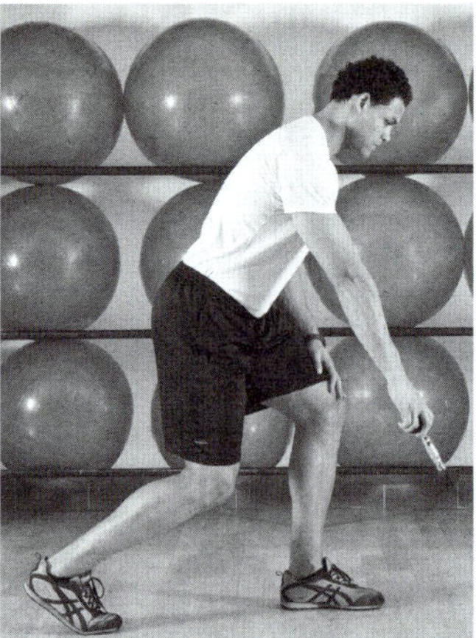

Reps: 10 per side
Sets: 1
Intensity: Light
Tempo: Slow and controlled
Rest: No rest needed

Starting position: Stand up straight with your feet together. Hold a 1- to 3-pound weight in your right hand with one end of the weight hanging down toward the floor.

Movement: Extend your right leg straight back and press the right heel toward the floor, bending your left knee slightly. Slowly rock your body forward and back, allowing the weight to swing gently like a pendulum. Finish all reps, then switch position and repeat with the weight in your left hand. This completes one set.

Tips and techniques:

- Maintain a neutral spine, and keep your shoulders down and back.
- Slant your whole body forward by hinging from the ankles.
- Rock back and forth, lifting the heel of the back leg and then the toe of the front leg.

Too hard? Perform the exercise while seated, or try it standing with no weight.

Too easy? Make a larger arc as you swing the weight like a pendulum.

3 | Strengthening: **Wall push-up with stability ball**

Reps: 10
Sets: 1–3
Intensity: Moderate
Tempo: 3-1-3
Rest: 30–90 seconds between sets

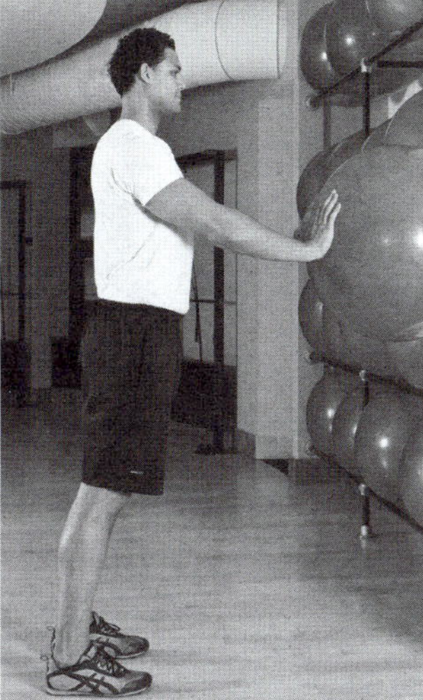

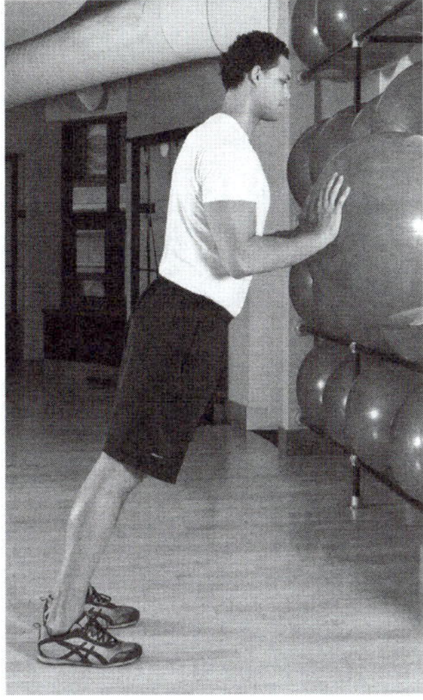

Starting position: Facing a wall, stand up straight to position a stability ball against the wall at shoulder height. Your arms should be extended at chest height with your palms against the ball, fingertips pointing toward the ceiling.

Movement: Slowly bend your elbows to lower your upper body toward the ball, keeping a straight line from head to heel. Pause, then slowly push away from the ball to return to the starting position. This is one rep.

Tips and techniques:

- Keep your fingertips no higher than shoulder level.
- Keep your elbows close to your sides as you bend them.
- Throughout the movement, maintain neutral alignment from head to toe, with your shoulders down and back.

Too hard? Try the wall push-up without the stability ball.
Too easy? After you lower your body toward the ball, hold the position for a count of eight. Then slowly push away from the ball to return to the starting position.

4 | Strengthening: **Standing internal and external rotation**

Reps: 10 of each step per side
Sets: 1–3
Intensity: Moderate to hard
Tempo: 3-1-3
Rest: 30–90 seconds between sets

Starting position: Anchor the resistance tubing to a door at waist level. Stand with your feet hip-width apart. Grasp one handle of the tubing in your right hand with your thumb pointed at the ceiling and your elbow firmly pinning a rolled-up hand towel at your side. Turn your body so that your right side faces the door, keeping tension on the tubing throughout the exercise.

Movement: This is a two-step exercise. **Step 1:** Keep your wrist firm as you slowly pull the band in toward your belly button like a door closing. Pause, then slowly return to the starting position. Finish all reps. **Step 2:** Switch hands so that you are grasping the handle with your left hand across your waist, knuckles near your belly button, and your left elbow pinning the hand towel at your side. (If necessary, adjust the tension on the resistance tubing by moving a bit closer to or farther away from the door.) Keep your wrist firm as you slowly pull the tubing outward like a door opening. Pause, then slowly return to the starting position. Finish all reps. Turn your body so that your left side faces the door and repeat both steps. This completes one set.

Tips and techniques:

- Maintain neutral posture, with your shoulders down and back.
- Note that the motion should come from the shoulder joint only. Hips should remain stationary at all times.
- Maintain a firm, neutral wrist.

Too hard? Use lighter resistance tubing.
Too easy? Use heavier resistance tubing.

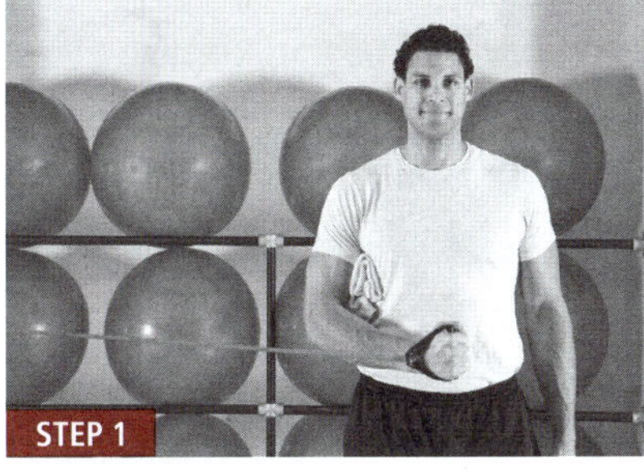
STEP 1

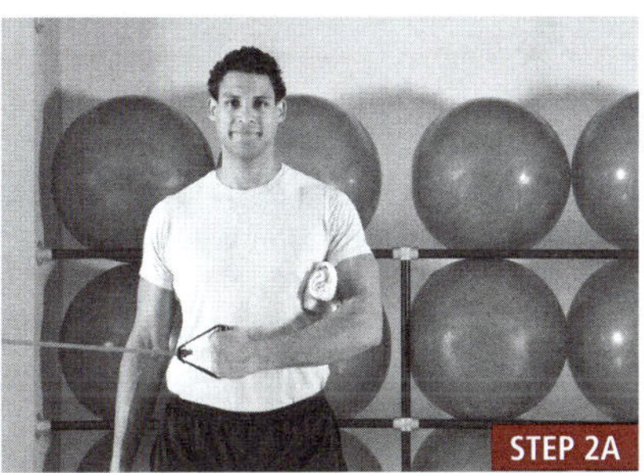
STEP 2A

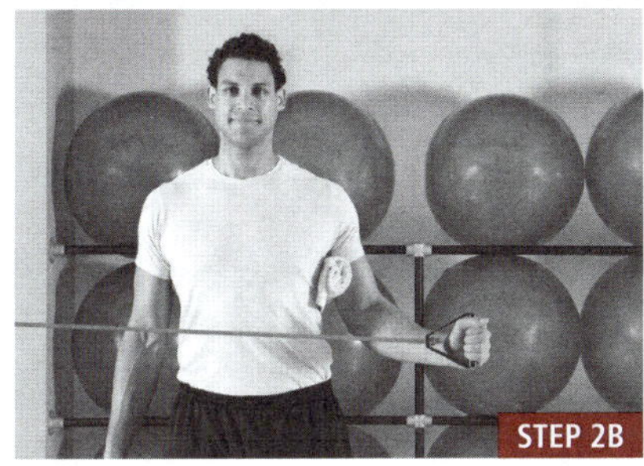
STEP 2B

5 | Strengthening: **Standing V-raise**

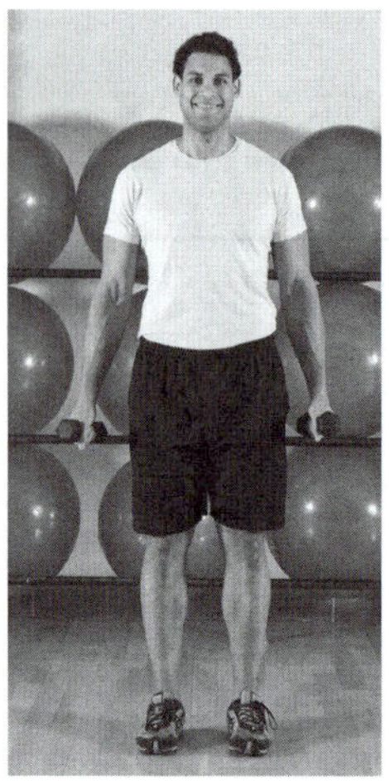
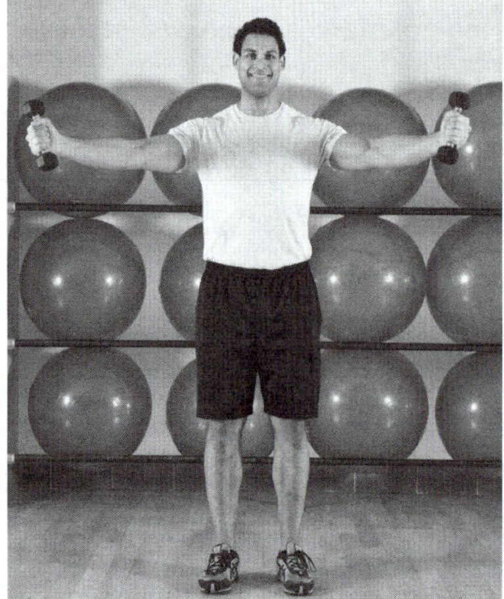

Reps: 10
Sets: 1–3
Intensity: Moderate

Tempo: 3-1-3
Rest: 30–90 seconds between sets

Starting position: Stand up straight holding 1- to 3-pound weights with your hands at your sides, thumbs facing forward. Position your feet hip-width apart.

Movement: Squeeze your shoulder blades together while you slowly lift your arms, creating a V as you raise the weights. Go no higher than your shoulders. Pause, then slowly return to the starting position. This is one rep.

Tips and techniques:

- Keep your wrists firm, maintaining a straight line from your elbow to your knuckles, and elbows soft (not locked) throughout the movement.
- Maintain neutral posture, with your shoulders down and back.
- Exhale as you lift.

Too hard? Use a lighter weight.
Too easy? Use a heavier weight.

6 | Strengthening: **Standing row**

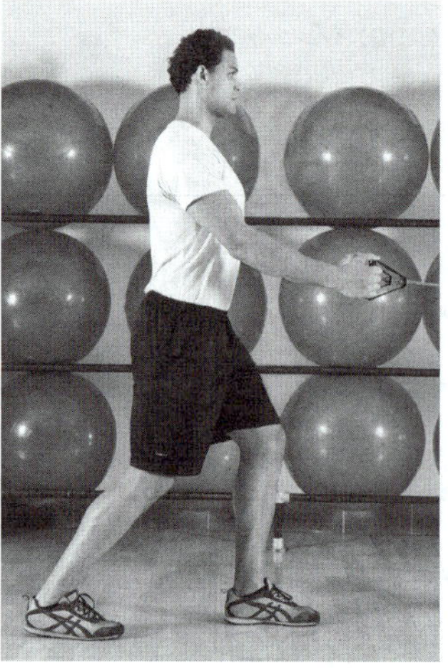
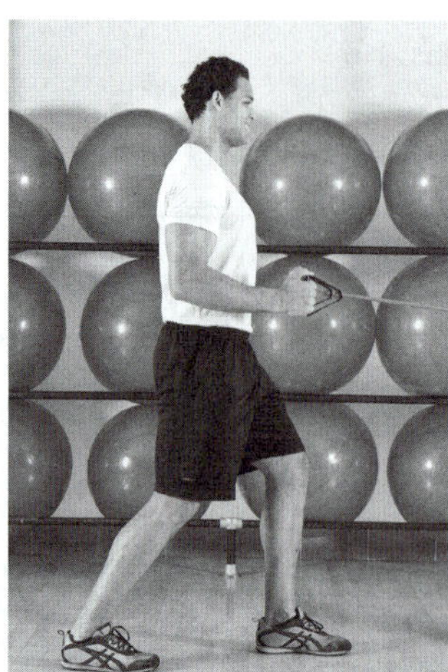

Reps: 10
Sets: 1–3
Intensity: Moderate

Tempo: 3-1-3
Rest: 30–90 seconds between sets

Starting position: Anchor the resistance tubing to a door at chest height. Stand up straight facing the door with your feet together. Stand far enough away from the door to put tension on the tubing as you hold the handles with your arms extended. Extend your right leg straight back and press the right heel toward the floor, bending both knees slightly.

Movement: Squeeze your shoulder blades together. Slowly bend your arms and pull back. Keep your elbows close to your ribs and pointing toward the back wall. Pause, then slowly return to the starting position. This is one rep.

Tips and techniques:

- Maintain neutral posture, with your shoulders down and back and your wrists firm.
- Exhale as you pull.

Too hard? Use lighter resistance tubing.
Too easy? Use heavier resistance tubing.

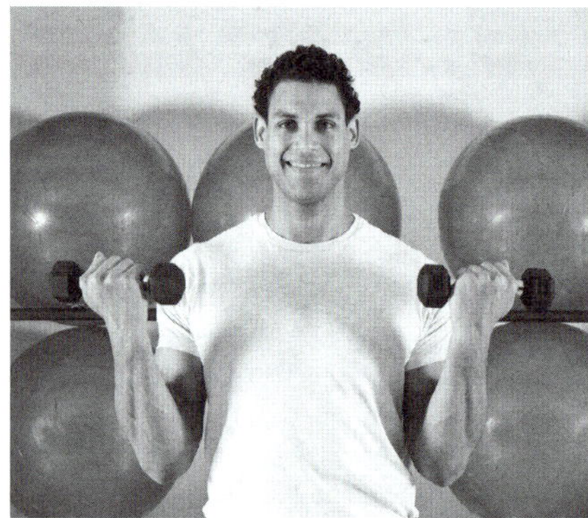

7 | Strengthening: **Biceps curl**

Reps: 10
Sets: 1–3
Intensity: Light to moderate

Tempo: 3-1-3
Rest: 30–90 seconds between sets

Starting position: Stand up straight with your feet hip-width apart, holding 1- to 3-pound weights at your side with your palms facing forward.

Movement: Slowly bend your elbows to lift the weights up to the front of your shoulders. Exhale as you lift. Pause. Slowly lower them to the starting position. This is one rep.

Tips and techniques:

- Keep your shoulders still, down, and back.
- Keep your wrists neutral and your elbows stationary at the sides of your ribs throughout the movement.

Too hard? Use lighter weights.
Too easy? Use heavier weights.

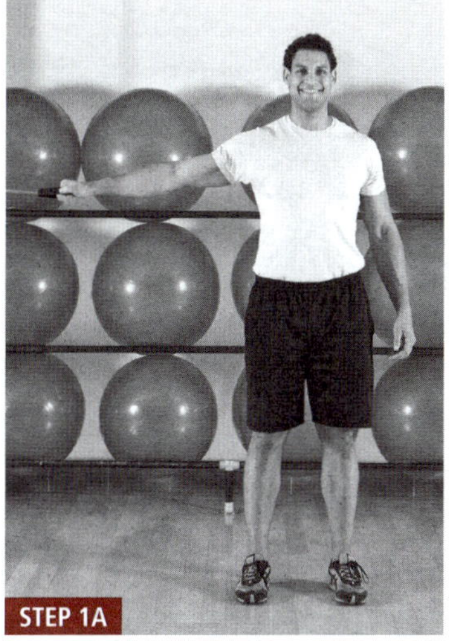
STEP 1A

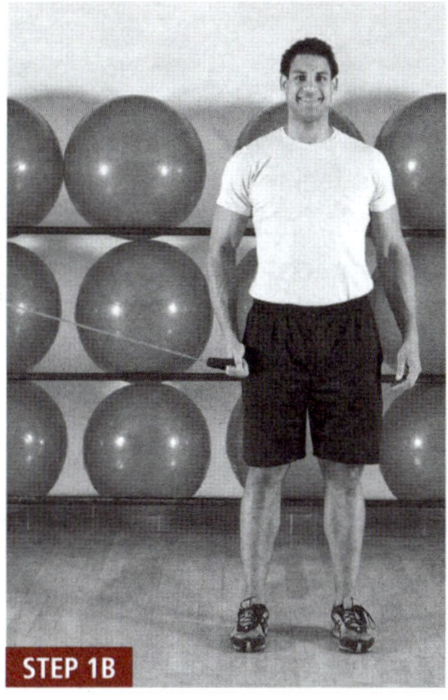
STEP 1B

STEP 2A

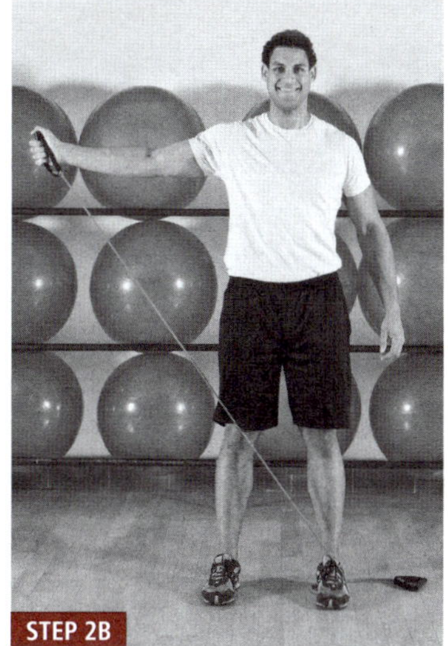
STEP 2B

8 | Strengthening: **Diagonals**

Reps: 10 of each step per side
Sets: 1–3
Intensity: Moderate
Tempo: 3-1-3
Rest: 30–90 seconds between sets

Starting position: Anchor resistance tubing to a door at chest level. Stand with your right side to the door. Position your legs hip-width apart, chest up, and shoulders down and back. Grasp the handle of the tubing horizontally in your right hand with your arm held out straight just below shoulder height. Keep tension on the tubing throughout the exercise.

Movement: This is a two-step exercise. **Step 1:** Keeping your wrist firm and arm straight, slowly pull your right arm down toward your right hip. Pause, then slowly return to the starting position. Finish all reps, then stand with your left side to the door and repeat, grasping the handle in your left hand.
Step 2: Anchor the resistance tubing to the floor with your left foot. Hold the handle with your right hand near your left hip, thumb toward the wall. Keeping your wrist firm, slowly lift your right hand up on a diagonal to shoulder height. Pause, then slowly bring your right hand back to your left hip. Finish all reps with the right arm before anchoring the tubing under your right foot and repeating with your left arm. This completes one set.

Tips and techniques:

- You may need to use lighter resistance tubing on this exercise to complete the movement with good form and ease.
- Keep your wrist firm and your shoulders down and back.
- Exhale as you pull.

Too hard? Use lighter resistance tubing.
Too easy? Use heavier resistance tubing.

9 | Stretching: **Shoulder stretch**

Reps: 3–4 per side
Sets: 1
Intensity: Light
Hold: 10–30 seconds
Rest: No rest needed

Starting position: Stand with your feet hip-width apart. Put your left hand on your right shoulder. Cup your left elbow with your right hand.

Movement: Roll your shoulders down and back as you gently pull your left elbow across your chest. Hold. Return to the starting position. Finish all reps, then repeat on the other side. This completes one set.

Tips and techniques:

- Stretch to the point of mild tension, not pain.
- Keep your shoulders down and back.
- Breathe comfortably.

Too hard? Stretch only as far as is comfortable.
Too easy? Repeat the stretch several times during the day.

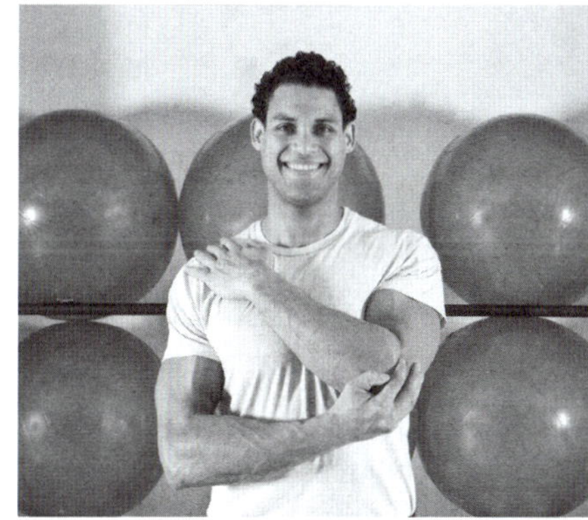

10 | Stretching: **Wall climb**

Reps: 3–4 of each step per side
Sets: 1
Intensity: Light to moderate
Hold: 10–30 seconds
Rest: No rest needed

Starting position: Stand up straight facing a wall.

Movement: This is a two-part exercise. **Step 1:** Extend your right arm with your elbow soft (not locked) and place your hand on the wall at shoulder height. Slowly walk your fingers upward, stepping in toward the wall as your hand climbs higher. Stop when you feel mild tension. Hold. Slowly walk your fingers back down the wall and return to the starting position. Finish all reps.
Step 2: Turn so that your right side faces the wall. Extend your right arm with your elbow soft (not locked) and place your hand on the wall at shoulder height. Slowly walk your fingers upward, stepping in toward the wall as your hand climbs higher. Stop when you feel mild tension. Hold. Slowly walk your fingers back down the wall and return to the starting position. Finish all reps. Repeat both steps using your left hand. This completes one set.

Tips and techniques:

- Stretch to the point of mild tension, not pain.
- Progress slowly toward the goal of bringing your body right next to the wall.
- Breathe comfortably.

Too hard? Place your hand on the wall below shoulder height and go only as high as is comfortable.

Too easy? Repeat the stretch several times throughout the day.

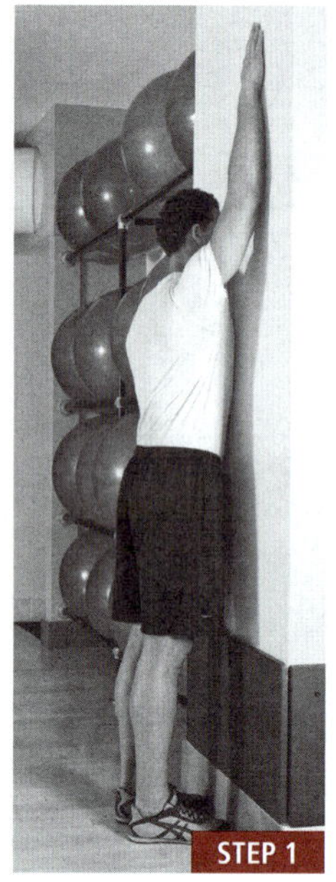
STEP 1

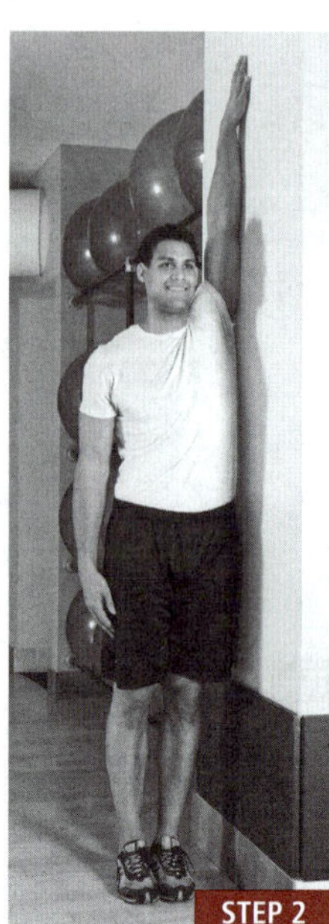
STEP 2

11 | Stretching: **Shoulder stretch with internal rotation**

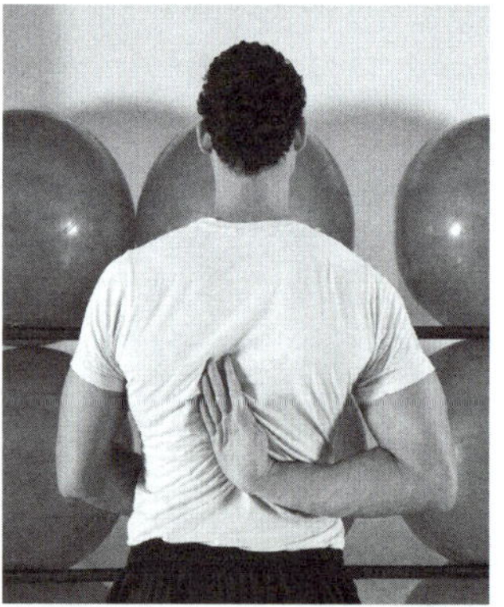

Reps: 3–4 per side
Sets: 1
Intensity: Moderate
Hold: 10–30 seconds
Rest: No rest needed

Starting position: Stand up straight with your feet hip-width apart and your hands by your sides.

Movement: Place the back of your right hand against the small of your back at your waist. Your fingers should be pointing up. Slowly slide your right hand farther up your back as high as you can. Hold. Finish all reps, then repeat with your left hand. This completes one set.

Tips and techniques:

- Stretch to the point of mild tension, not pain.
- Maintain neutral posture, with your shoulders down and back.
- Breathe comfortably.

Too hard? Make your movement smaller.

Too easy? Repeat the stretch several times during the day.

12 | Stretching: **Chest stretch**

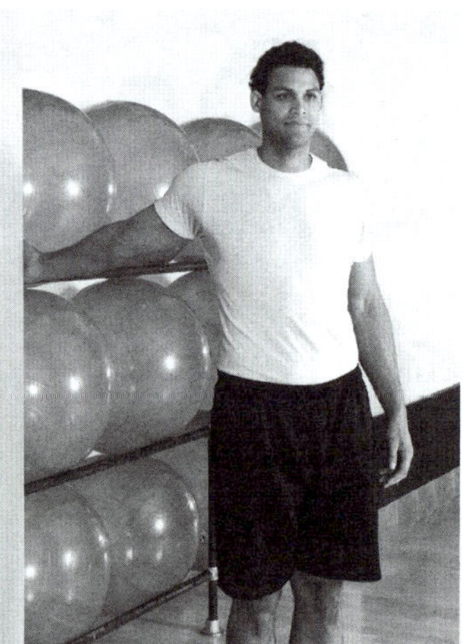

Reps: 3–4 per side
Sets: 1
Intensity: Light to moderate
Hold: 10–30 seconds
Rest: No rest needed

Starting position: Stand alongside a doorway. Extend your right arm and put your right hand on the edge of the door frame slightly below shoulder level, palm facing forward and touching the door frame. Keep your shoulders down and back.

Movement: Slowly turn your body to the left, away from the door frame, until you feel the stretch in your chest and shoulder. Hold. Return to the starting position. Finish all reps, then repeat on the opposite side. This completes one set.

Tips and techniques:

- Stretch to the point of mild tension, not pain.
- Breathe comfortably.

Too hard? Make your movement smaller.

Too easy? Repeat the stretch several times during the day.

Wrist and elbow mini-workout

If you're an avid athlete sidelined by tennis elbow or golfer's elbow, or an office athlete wincing from job-related repetitive motions, this workout can get you back in the game by enhancing flexibility and strengthening supporting muscles. We recommend performing the full workout two to three times a week.

One additional easy exercise—squeezing a rubber ball 30 times at a slow, controlled pace—needs no illustration and can be practiced daily to improve your grip. The squishier the ball, the easier the workout, so choose a firmer rubber ball when you're ready for more of a challenge. If you have arthritis, try putting your hands in warm water while squeezing the ball.

Equipment: Hand weights (1 to 3 pounds), sturdy chair, rubber ball.

1 | Warming up and stretching: **Wrist circle warm-up**

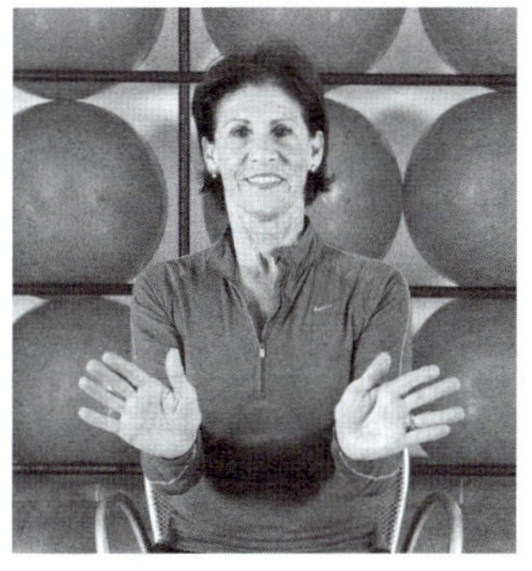

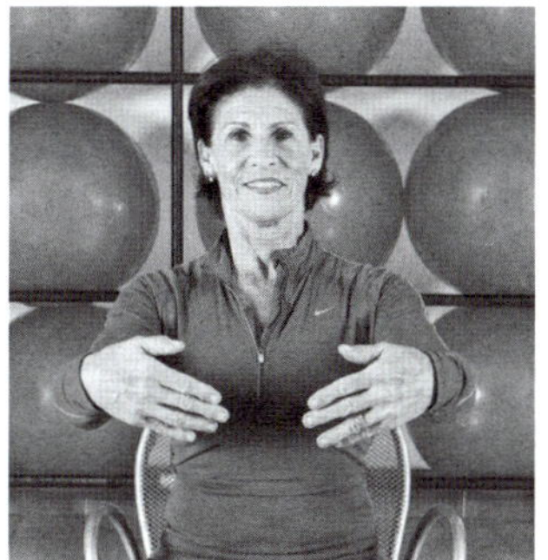

Reps: 10 in each direction
Sets: 1–3
Intensity: Light
Tempo: Slow and controlled
Rest: No rest needed

Starting position: Sit in a chair or stand up straight.

Movement: Slowly circle your wrists 10 times in one direction, then 10 times in the other direction. This completes one set.

Tips and techniques:

- Maintain neutral posture, with your shoulders down and back.
- Breathe comfortably.

Too hard? Make smaller circles.

Too easy? Repeat the warm-up several times throughout the day.

2 | Warming up and stretching: **Wrist stretch**

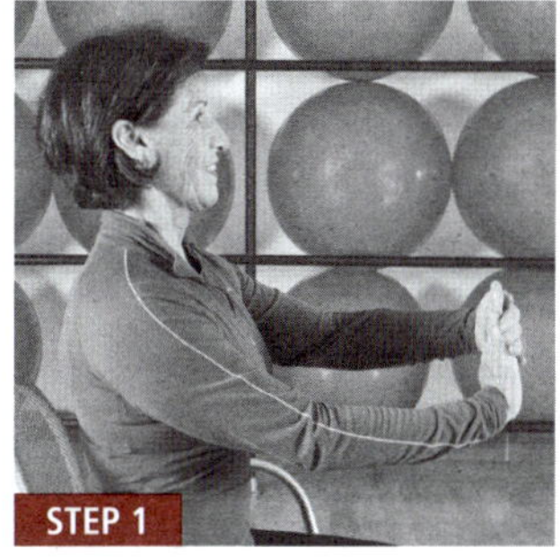
STEP 1

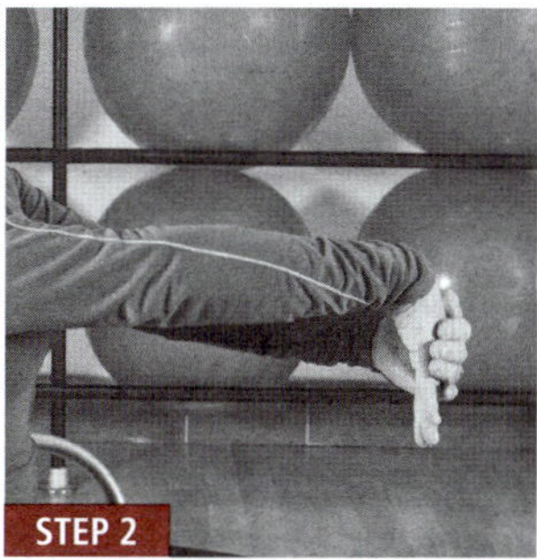
STEP 2

Reps: 3–4 per side
Sets: 1
Intensity: Light
Hold: 10–30 seconds
Rest: No rest needed

Starting position: Sit in a chair with your right arm and hand extended in front of you with the palm down, facing the floor.

Movement: This is a two-step exercise. **Step 1:** Point the fingers of your right hand toward the ceiling. Place the palm of your left hand in front of your right hand. Gently press your left hand against the palm and fingers of your right hand to increase the stretch, stopping if you feel any pain. Hold. Return to the starting position. **Step 2:** Bend your right hand forward at the wrist, pointing your fingers downward into a fully flexed position. Cup the back of your right hand with your left hand. Gently press downward with your left hand to increase the stretch, stopping if you feel any pain. Hold. Finish all reps, then switch arms and repeat both steps on your left hand. This completes one set.

Tips and techniques:

- Stretch to the point of mild tension, not pain.
- Maintain neutral posture, with your shoulders down and back.
- Breathe comfortably.

Too hard? Press more gently to limit the range of motion.

Too easy? Repeat the stretch several times throughout the day.

3 | Warming up and stretching: **Wrist flexion and extension**

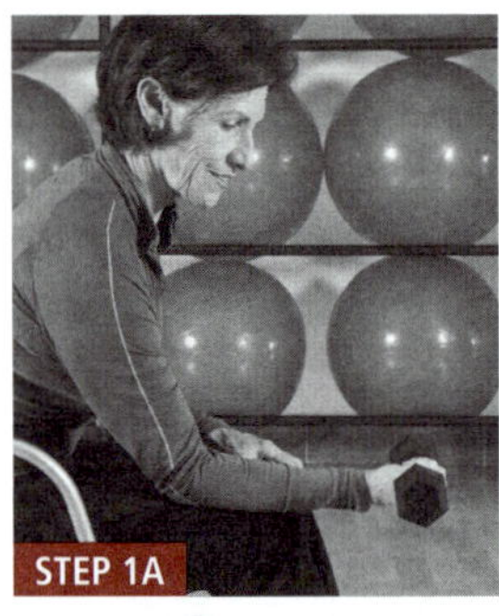
STEP 1A

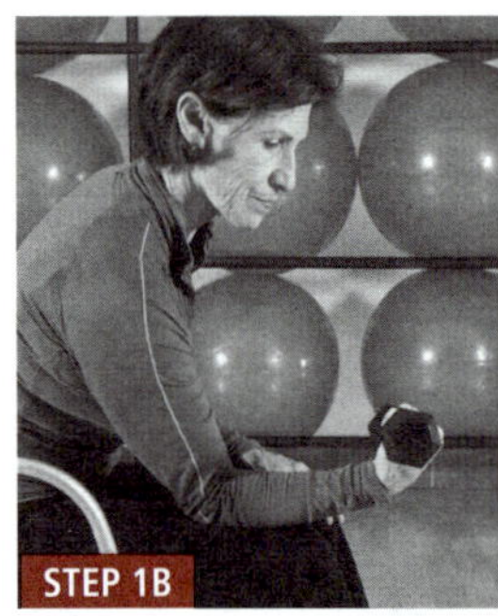
STEP 1B

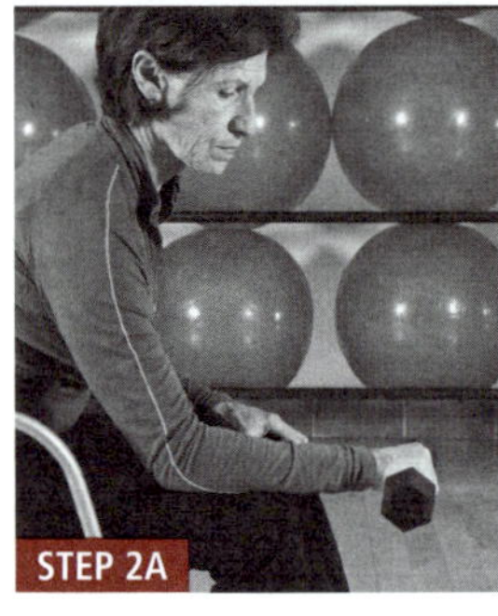
STEP 2A

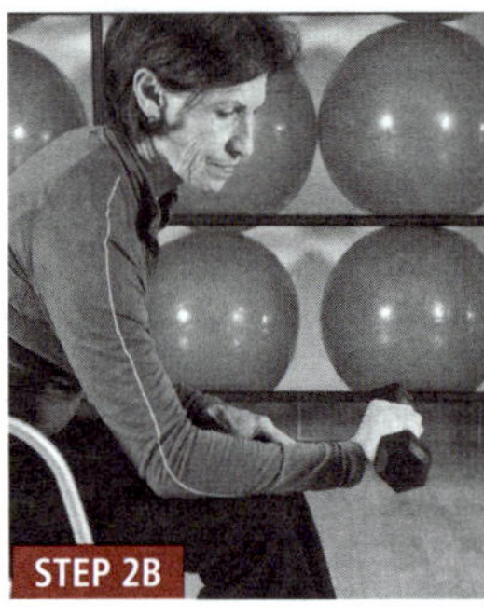
STEP 2B

Reps: 10 of each step per side
Sets: 1–3
Intensity: Light
Tempo: 3-1-3
Rest: 30–90 seconds between sets

Starting position: Sit in a chair holding a 1-pound weight in your right hand, palm facing up and wrist neutral. Lean forward, bending at the hip, and place the back of your right forearm on your thigh.

Movement: This is a two-step exercise. **Step 1:** Slowly curl your right hand upward. Pause, then slowly return to the starting position so that your wrist is neutral. Finish all reps, then repeat with your left hand holding the weight. **Step 2:** Reverse the exercise. Hold the light weight in your right hand, palm facing down, wrist neutral, and forearm supported on your thigh. Slowly bend your wrist backward to lift up the weight. Pause, and slowly return to the neutral wrist position. Finish all reps, then repeat with your left hand holding the weight. This completes one set.

Tips and techniques:

- Maintain a neutral spine, with your shoulders down and back.
- Be sure to return to a neutral wrist at the beginning and end of each rep.
- Breathe comfortably, exhaling as you lift.

Too hard? Use a lighter weight or no weight.
Too easy? Use a heavier weight.

4 | Warming up and stretching: **Palm up, palm down**

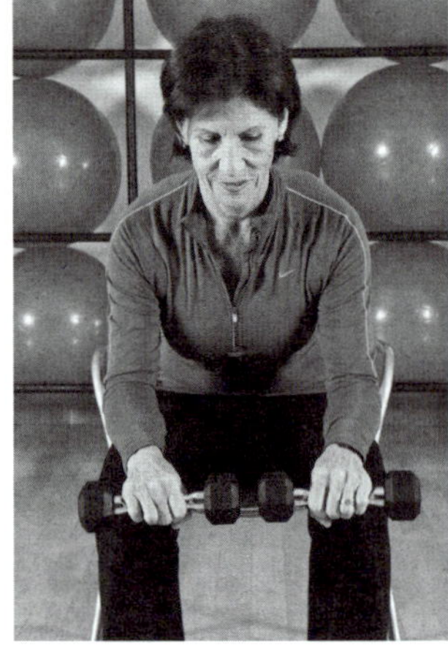

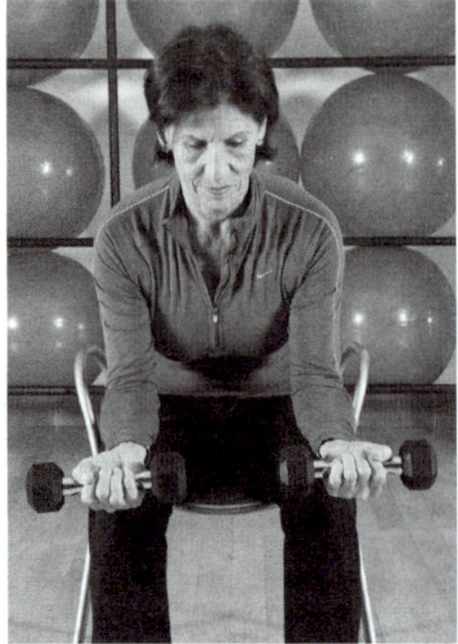

Reps: 10
Sets: 1–3
Intensity: Light
Tempo: 3-1-3
Rest: 30–90 seconds between sets

Starting position: Sit in a chair holding a 1-pound weight in each hand with your elbows slightly bent and your palms facing the floor. Your wrists should be neutral.

Movement: Slowly turn your hands over until your palms face the ceiling. Pause, then slowly return to the starting position. This is one rep.

Tips and techniques:

- Maintain a neutral spine, with your shoulders down and back.
- Keep your wrists neutral throughout the movement.
- Breathe comfortably.

Too hard? Use lighter weights or no weights.
Too easy? Use heavier weights.